Operation...

Pull Your Own Weight!

A Radically Simple, User Friendly, Preventative Solution To The Childhood Obesity Epidemic!

Dedicated to IMMUNIZING kids against obesity naturally, without resorting to pills, shots, surgery, or special diets!

Copyright Notices

Legal Notices

A Bad Joke That Makes A Point...

Have you heard the following joke?

Did you ever notice when geese are flying overhead in their V formation, that one side of the V is always a little longer than the other? Do you know why?

Now you allow the person being questioned time to percolate on the answer, eyes to the ceiling, flipping through their mental Rolodex trying to come up with an answer that's clever or sophisticated in some way. When they give up, you tell deliver the punch line...

It's because there are more geese on one side of the V than the other!!!

OK, I can see the eyes rolling now, and I hear all the comments about this being such a stupid joke, etc. But I tell it for a purpose. At the heart of this joke is the presumption that the person being questioned will look high and low for a clever answer, while overlooking the one blatantly obvious answer that's staring 'em right in the face.

Much like this bad joke, I contend that the answer to the childhood obesity epidemic in this country and around the world is so blatantly obvious that we're overlooking it in an effort to come up with more clever, or sophisticated, high tech solutions in this age of high tech everything. Read on and see if you agree.

Table of Contents

Dedication: Babcock

The Appendix

Babcock...

"Can you remember a spring day in your thirteenth year? A seductive breeze, a few white clouds sketched by a careless artist, the sun striking maddening smells from the moist earth and encouraging unaccustomed pulses in various parts of your body.

It was just such a day in 1972, on a late-morning walk in a small Virginia town, that I came across a group of some thirty-five or forty thirteen-year-olds sitting on a grassy bank. I was on a lecture tour, summoned from my motel by the sight and smell of April blossoms.

Standing in front of boys and girls was a taut-muscled young man in gym shoes, gym pants, a white T-shirt, a crew cut, a whistle, and a clipboard. Next to the young man, like a guillotine in the sunlight, was a chinning bar. I stopped to observe the scene.

The man looked at his clipboard. 'Babcock' he called.

There was a stir among the boys and girls. One of them rose and made his way to the chinning bar: Babcock the classic fat boy.

Shoulders slumped, he stood beneath the bar. 'I can't,' he said.

'You can try,' the man with the clipboard said.

Babcock reached up with both hands, touched the bar limply –just that-and walked away, his eyes downcast, as all the boys and girls watched, seeming to share in his shame.

I also walked on, flushed with anger. Beneath the anger, I sensed something tentative and hurt. The incident seemed to touch an area of my past that I had conveniently forgotten. The day was so lovely-no time to explore painful areas. I started thinking about other things.

But Babcock was not to let me off so easily. The vignette kept replaying itself in my mind. I was fascinated by the way the fat boy walked to the chin up bar, waddling slightly but moving fast as if eager to have it done with; his condemned stance beneath the bar, the minimal, symbolic touch of his hands on the metal; his utter resignation as he walked away, his head bobbing from side to side.

Again and again, Babcock rose, walked to the bar, stood there, touched the bar, walked off. The scene took on the quality of a Greek drama. The man with the clipboard became the stern-visaged god who devises tests for us, then sends us on without mercy to our respective fates. The boys and girls took the part of the chorus, by their silence condemning the unworthy, and yet by the same silence, expressing their own uneasiness and shame."

…From George Leonard's Classic Book, *The Ultimate Athlete*

So What Can We Do For Babcock?

Well, as it turns out, in the Chicago area Babcock represents at least 23% of all kids under the age of seven. Nationwide, it's more than 10%. And if you use the pull up bar as your acid test, the figures actually grow dramatically worse because upper body weakness also comes into play.

The question then for the remainder of this book is…how can we help the Babcocks across the country? *What can we do to give them the strength and the confidence required to…*

- *set a goal,*

- *get a couple workouts in each week for a prescribed period of time,*
- *eat right,*
- *get sufficient rest,*
- *avoid negative habits including tobacco, alcohol, and drugs,*
- *grab hold of the damn pull up bar*
- *and show the world that they can do it too?*
- That's the specific challenge that motivates rest of this book.

Introduction
The Simple Solution To Childhood Obesity That Doesn't Require A Book

Here, in a nutshell, is the conceptual foundation for this simple, natural, and functional solution to the childhood obesity epidemic in this country. And if you understand it, you can probably figure out how to proceed to a successful end without ever reading the remainder of this book. Check it out.

Wall A, Wall B Story

Go into any school gym in the country and ask all the students who can perform at least one pull up to stand by wall A, and all those who can't to stand by wall B. What you'll then see is what I call The Great Fitness Divide, with all the relatively lean and strong students on wall A, and all the relatively overweight and weak students on wall B.

My conclusion? Start very young (grades K, 1, or 2) before most kids have a chance to gain too much excess weight, and teach them to be able to perform pull ups. Then make them understand that if they maintain their _ability to perform pull ups_, they'll always be relatively lean and strong, and they'll never be much overweight and weak, or experience all the related problems. Isn't it about time to teach all kids from sea to shining sea to Pull Their Own Weight?

The Book Is Unnecessary, But...

I want to say right up front that the case for implementing this strategy can, and has been made many times in the form of short essays or a stand alone articles. You don't need to read an entire book to understand it. However since I and others have written a number of pieces on the subject, attacking and explaining it from various perspectives, I contend that a collection of these essays and articles will make an interesting and informative book for parents, educators, and health professionals who are tired of waiting for the experts to come up with a magic pill, and who want to stop childhood obesity in its tracks now with a simple and naturalistic solution...the ability to perform pull ups.

Because of the nature of the book, there will be some repetition and overlap in the following chapters. But if you read through them, I suggest that you'll come out the other end with a thorough and practical understanding of this simple, functional solution to the childhood obesity epidemic that you can implement with your own kids, or students with little time, expense, or hassle.

A Parent Volunteer Speaks Out on Behalf of Operation Pull Your Own Weight

Re: The Pull Your Own Weight Program

To Whom It May Concern:

I began working as a volunteer with the Pull Your Own Weight Program in February of this year. Within a couple of weeks *I found myself so enthused and engrossed in it that my volunteer time doubled.*

The best aspect of the Pull Your Own Weight Program is the holistic approach it entails. It covers the social, psychological, and the physical needs of the individual.

The children are able to perform in this program no matter what their age, size, or economic background is. *They participate enthusiastically, often asking to do more than my schedule allows time for.* The sense of accomplishment and pride is apparent in their faces as they learn more and more discipline in the physical and mental challenges of Pull Your Own Weight.

Psychologically this program encourages strength of mind and a sense of self-esteem that one usually associates with a martial arts program. *Weekly I watch these children learn to challenge themselves, and <u>never once</u> have I seen this turn into a competition between peers.* These children all have a sense of giving when it comes to urging and cheering on their classmates.

The students who take part in this program show a high degree of self initiative, striving to always better their last score. *<u>They begin to understand</u> that in many things, the only obstacle between them and success is their own attitude and effort.* And through this program they learn to push themselves towards realistic goals.

The practical steps, objectives, and possibilities of attainment are all geared towards creating a situation in which *the child can generate his or her own limits and <u>see them become fact</u>* long before the interest fades. And so the interest never does diminish, because for each new level reached, the children find a new one to attempt.

Physically these children become stronger each time they use the methods offered them. They can *<u>see their own strength blossom</u> in a rapid and understandable manner.* And while they focus mainly on arm strength, they eventually notice that *the strength extends to the whole child.*

The program *requires so little for the achievements produced* that it is definitely something that should be recommended for all schools.

I urge any and all support for such a rewarding project as The Pull Your Own Weight Program. It encourages unity, self-esteem, and strength. *Very few programs offer so much at one time*. And the message entailed in the name itself is one that can be recognized and hailed by everyone.

Sincerely,

Devoura Lee Cooks
Jefferson Elementary School
Davenport, IA
March 7, 1991

Mother Nature Defines Fitness In Functional, Not Cosmetic Terms

In nature, out in the wild, animals who are overweight (unfit) are not tolerated, and obesity just can't happen. If an antelope for example, gains a few extra pounds, he gets one step slower and becomes easy prey for Mamma lion. If Mamma lion picks up a few extra pounds, she won't catch up to the antelope. As the result she'll naturally miss a few meals, eventually sheds the excess weight, and she'll be back in the hunt.

Moving a little closer to home, if a squirrel picks up extra weight, he'll be unable to climb trees or leap from limb to limb with total abandon. He may even miss, fall, and become a tasty treat for the local cat. And if a robin in your backyard picks up a little extra luggage, she'll have a harder time getting off the ground and into flight. At that point the local cat might just make a meal out of her as well.

I could go on and on here, but I'm sure you see the point that, out in the wild (even the suburban wilderness), where survival depends on an animal's ability to avoid a predator, or a predator's ability to catch up to its prey, there's simply zero tolerance for excess body weight if an animal wants to continue breathing.

The Lone Exception to Mother Nature's Ironclad Rule

The only instance in with Mother Nature temporarily tolerates excess weight is in animals that hibernate for a certain period of the year. The bear for example, is an animal who, before going into hibernation takes on extra calories, packs on an extra layer of fat, and then he goes to sleep for several months, eating nothing. He's effectively living off of the stored fat in his system. But when he awakes in the spring, the excess weight will be gone, and he's back in the position of having to earn his daily meals by catching up with his prey every day, and his excess weight will be gone for the season.

Obesity and Domestication

Other than that, excess weight is found only in domesticated animals. That is to say you'll find fat pigs, and hefty heifers out on the farm. You'll see fat dogs and occasionally even fat cats who have become so domesticated and dependent on their human masters that they've fattened up to the point of being physically incapable of surviving in the wild. Animals that don't have to physically earn their daily bread, or physically avoid being turned into someone else's daily bread, have the option of becoming overweight. But any animal that has to catch his prey, or run from a predator, can ill afford the luxury of being overweight.

And What About Our Closest Ancestor?

Before moving on to the domesticated human species let's take a quick look at man's closest cousin, the monkey (or the gorilla). In fact let me ask, can you even imagine seeing a fat monkey or gorilla out in the wild? If a monkey gains much weight, climbing trees with the greatest of ease, and swinging from limb to limb Tarzan style, becomes a physical impossibility. The result? No fat monkeys in the jungle!

What Can We Learn From Mother Nature?

So Mother Nature basically defines fitness (or the lack of it) in functional terms, not in cosmetic terms. That is to say, she wants to know what you can do with your body, not what do you look like? On the other hand it's also no secret that there's a definite sense of beauty found in a well developed, fully functioning, and confident human physique, and in many cultures, including the ancient Greeks, they celebrated it.

But in nature it's function first and beauty second, not the other way around. With all that said, let's ask what can modern, domesticated man learn from Mother Nature, and how can we apply this knowledge to the childhood obesity epidemic sitting out on our front doorstep? Let's talk about that right now.

The Peace Corps' Solution To Obesity

In light of our previous comments about Mother Nature and her intolerance for obesity at almost any level, one solution to the obesity problem would be to chuck the modern lifestyle that encourages poor eating habits and inactivity, and go back into the wild. It's not as if that has not been done before. Certain kinds of scientists do it on a regular basis in order to study nature in various ways.

I have a good friend who volunteered for the Peace Corps and served a year in Africa (Gambia to be precise) and he confirmed that overeating and lack of physical exercise are non-existent in the Gambian tribal cultures where he lived for a year. This guy, by the way was trim when he left, and even trimmer when he came back. There are also missionaries who represent various church groups who go into the third world, and who actually benefit physically from the lack of junk food and television sets.

Answer This Simple Question

But presuming that you're not an Indiana Jones kind of scientist, or that you're not the missionary type, and the Peace Corps just doesn't fit into the schedule right now, what are your naturalistic options here in domestic captivity? In order to best answer that question let me pose another question. How many activities can you make the following statement about? I CAN'T BE OVERWEIGHT AS LONG AS I CAN STILL DO _____! Use your imagination and see what you can come up with.

Three Easy To See Examples...

There are lots of answers to that question. How about running fast or running long? I mean people who are overweight can't run fast or long right? Let's test the statement and see if it makes sense? I can't be overweight as long as I can still run fast or run long. Does that work for you? It sure does for me. Let's try another one.

How about jumping high or long? I know people who can get way off the floor on a vertical jump test. These same people can jump lengthwise as well. But those who can perform these feats are definitely not overweight. So here we go again...I can't be overweight as long as I can still jump high or jump long. Another winner, right?

22

Let's try one more to make sure we have it straight. How about climbing on climbing walls, or on the sides of mountains? I've seen lots of photos of climbers and I've never seen one who's carrying any excess weight. So, I can't be overweight as long as I can still climb the wall or the mountain. That's one more in the winner's circle, right?

So what kinds of conclusions can we draw from these observations that are pertinent to the childhood obesity issue? Would you agree with me if I said "if a child learns to run fast or long, climb a wall or the side of a mountain, or jump high or long, you can safely bet on the fact that they will not be overweight?" It's really quite simple. Where you have functional ability, whether it's in the wilds of darkest Africa or in the suburbs of Chicago, you will find no instances of overweight/obesity.

But My Kid's A Musician Not An Athlete...

But you say "Wait a minute. What if I live in the city and my children don't have the time, the opportunity, or the desire to learn to run, jump, or climb? What if my kids are more into music or drama or academics? Aren't there any naturalistic, functional options for them to choose from?" The answer is...there sure are. Let's have a look.

Dips On The Parallel Or Monkey Bars

Dips are an exercise performed on parallel bars or monkey bars in which the participant starts in the up position (graphic A), lower yourself down into the down position (graphic B), and then push yourself back up again. The exercise works the chest and the triceps primarily, and it's most often seen in gymnastic oriented activities. Dips are an exercise in which the entire body weight is the resistance factor and if you can do any of them the odds of being overweight are very minimal.

Dips, like all body weight exercises, pay for fat loss and for strength (muscle) gain. That means that if you improve your ability to do dips, you're either losing fat, gaining muscle, or both. Which is just another way of saying your body composition is improving and your percentage of body fat is going down. So let's give dips our little test right now. I can't be overweight if I can still do dips. This one works for me.

Hand Stand Push Ups

Another good example is an exercise known as handstand push ups. As the name indicates, in this exercise you flip upside down and stand on your hands instead of your feet, and balance yourself. Then you lower yourself down, touch your nose to the floor, and push yourself back up into the starting position. (see the graphics)

The one factor that comes into play for this exercise is balance. You can be strong and lean, and have a poor sense of balance which undermines your ability to perform hand stand push ups. But other than that, the scenario works. This exercise pays for any performer to lose fat, gain strength, for body composition improvement, and a reduction in percentage of body fat. Shall we try our test? I can't be overweight as long as I can still do hand stand push ups. Absolutely true, right? It works once again.

Superman Push Ups

The third example I'd like to talk about is called the Superman Push Up, because when the participant is doing the exercise they look like Superman flying over Metropolis looking for Lex Luthor or some other super villain doing bad things to good people. All that aside, the participant performs this exercise with an exercise wheel in hand, starting in what is the conventional push up position. They roll the wheel out until they're stretched out (graphics) in the Superman position, and then roll back up into the starting position.

This exercise is very challenging to the core muscles (the abdominals and the lower back) and if done wrong it can cause lower back problems. However it definitely pays the participant to lose fat, gain strength, improve body composition, and reduce your percentage of body fat. As for the test, let's give it a try. If I can still do Superman Push Ups, I can't be overweight. Yep, that works again, doesn't it?

Sissy Squats

Sissy squats are basically leg extensions that use the participant's own body weight as the resistance. Blocking off the front of the ankles and the back of the knees, you lower yourself backwards until your thighs are parallel with the ground. If you bend at the waist this exercise is much easier than if you remain straight from the knees up…in other words if you avoid bending at the waist.

Sissy squats isolate the quadriceps and they pay for fat loss, strength gain, improved body composition, and reduced percentage of body fat. In other words sissy squats are not really for sissies, and if I can still do the most difficult variety of sissy squats, I can't be overweight? That's absolutely true.

Rope Climbing

The fourth example I want to talk about is Rope Climbing. If you're in school you may have seen this done in the recent past. If you're out of school you may have to recollect your days in gym class. Either way, if you can start at the bottom, climb to the top, and let yourself back down under control (avoiding a roper burn, which is the potential negative factor with this one), that's a pretty darn good trick.

The rope pays for fat loss, strength gain, improved body composition, and reduced percentage of body fat. And I can't be overweight as long as I can still climb a rope. The statement is absolutely true then about rope climbing, sissy squats, Superman push ups, hand stand push ups, and dips. If you can do any one of them, and maintain the ability, you are not now, and you never will be overweight. Now there's an interesting thought in the midst of an obesity epidemic, wouldn't you agree?

Any One of These Will Work For Any Body

I'm here to say that *any one of these exercises, alone and by themselves, could serve as a functional antidote to childhood obesity*, adolescent obesity, and adult obesity without a pill, without a health club membership, without a degree in Physical Education, and with hardly any time or expense to speak of. It's perfect for students who are into music, debate, art, and drama instead of sports and athletics. And they're all natural, something that

27

Mother Nature might expect of her own animal population out in the wild.

And Then There Are Pull Ups

Are there any other exercises that would immunize and vaccinate any human being, including all children, against being overweight? You could discover more if you really put your mind to it. But there's one more in particular that I want to mention because for my money it's the best example. But you're going to have to move on to the next chapter to discover everything I want to tell you about a wonderful little exercise called PULL UPS. Check it out…

What Inspired Me To Write A Book About The Simplest Antidote To Childhood Obesity On Earth

The biggest complaint I ever got on *Operation Pull Your Own Weight* was when Superintendent Peter Flynn said that it was generating more positive publicity for one school than all the rest (28 in all) of the district's schools combined. It was of course, a tongue in cheek criticism from Flynn that I gladly accepted as a compliment to the program, but it was certainly not enough to inspire me to write a book.

The one other criticism that I got on the program was from one physical educator who said that "it lacked the comprehensiveness of a sound fitness program." However, this well intended fellow was overlooking the fact that OPYOW was never intended to be a comprehensive fitness program. It was nothing more (and nothing less) than a simple, functional antidote to obesity that could be easily implemented by almost anyone for almost no money.

It was also very safe, took very little time, and as Dr. Flynn so eloquently pointed out, it generated boatloads of good ink for Jefferson School in Davenport, IA for four consecutive years. But even that failed to inspire me to write a book on the subject.

This Finally Inspired Me To Write A Book...

However, when I started reading story after story about our nation's childhood obesity epidemic in newspapers and magazines, and hearing about it on the radio, and seeing it on television, and the internet, my creative juices began flowing. I read that the federal government had earmarked MEGABUCK$$ to combat childhood obesity, which currently effects 10% of all kids nationally. The childhood obesity story was running in Time Magazine, on Oprah, and almost everywhere else in the modern media universe.

In short, childhood obesity was apparently growing like wildfire and creating a multi-billion dollar annual problem, yet nobody was talking about the one solution that every single gym teacher in the world already knows about. Now all that combined inspired me to write a book.

What's The Secret You Ask...

So, what exactly is this incredibly simple solution that's visible only to gym teachers you ask? It was the common observation (by the way, you don't have to be a gym teacher to recognize it) that kids who can do pull ups are never obese. On the other hand, kids who are obese can never do pull ups. Pull ups and obesity are mutually exclusive, and never found in the same person. They avoid one another like the plague.

The functional antidote to childhood obesity that lies at the center of *Operation Pull Your Own Weight* is the strategy that was used at Jefferson Elementary School in Davenport, IA to cost effectively (cheaply) teach kids at to develop the ability, and to love their "opportunity" to practice doing pull ups. You see, our kids (K-3) not only learned to do pull ups, but they also learned to take pride in their ability, and to look forward to doing them. They also learned that as long as they maintained their ability to do pull ups, they could never, ever be much overweight. Yes, you're are effectively immunized against obesity for life, as long as you continue to be able to do pull ups.

I'm Only Speculating, But...

I'm speculating here, but I'd be willing to bet that Jefferson Elementary is the only school in the history of the world where kids actually looked forward to the privilege of doing pull ups, and in the process became functionally immunized against obesity for the rest of their lives...if they chose to be. Yes, my new book, *Operation Pull Your Own*

31

Weight: A Radically Simple, User Friendly, Preventative Solution To The Childhood Obesity Epidemic That's Actively Stalking The World's Kids Today, explains the program in easily digestible terms so that anyone who is action oriented, and genuinely interested in making a significant dent in the childhood obesity epidemic, and generating boatloads of positive publicity in the process, can do so.

Who's The Target Audience?

Who's the book's intended audience you ask?

- The first audience is parents, because PYOW can easily be taught at home in less than ten minutes a week, with little to no related cost.

- The second audience is the professional physical educator whether you're in a school, a health club, a YM/WCA, a Boys and Girls Club, a Park District, or in a corporate wellness (this includes fire and police departments) setting.

- The third audience is educational administrators and school boards (including their public relations people) who want to generate some great press while resolving a real live problem.

- A fourth and final audience will be college and university level physical education classes, although they will most likely find the concept far too simplistic, and they'll overlook it's greatest strength…its sheer simplicity.

So if you fit into any one of these groups and are looking to take action, read on and discover how simple the solution to the childhood obesity epidemic can actually be. And once you make this discovery, follow it up with real live action, whether it's with your own kids at home, in your classroom at school, or in any one of the other settings that we've mentioned in this brief analysis. And don't forget to tell your local media what you're doing. If they are anything like the media in Davenport, IA they will be more than a little willing to cover positive news about kids, in almost any setting. Just go for it.

My Own Personal Qualifications

I can hear somebody asking "What qualifies you, Mr. Osbourne, to be prescribing any solution to this very serious national problem?" I will answer this challenge with the following comments. I'm an ex-physical education teacher who spent seventeen years in the profession before opting out and moving over to the private sector nine years ago. But for four of those seventeen years ('90 – '94) I was part of the largest "at risk grant" in the state of Iowa, and was, among other things, placed in charge of a special fitness based, self esteem program called *Operation Pull Your Own Weight (PYOW for short).*

The program was specifically designed to improve the self esteem, confidence, and the related performances (which includes just about everything) of all kindergarten through third grade students who attended Jefferson Elementary School in Davenport, IA, by showing them how to beat the odds of becoming overweight by helping them to learn to perform pull ups. Here's the basic logic behind Operation PYOW.

Presumption # 1: Fitness Improves Self Esteem

The program was based on four presumptions, the first being that a child who is physically lean and strong feels more confident than a child who is overweight and weak. At the time there was no specific research to substantiate this presumption. But since then there has been lots of research showing that kids who are overweight suffer from poor self esteem, and the low self esteem tends to discourage performance in many other aspects of their life as well.

Presumption # 2: Pull Ups... A Functional Acid Test

The second presumption of the PYOW program was that we could separate the strong and lean kids from the overweight kids by testing their ability to perform pull ups. In other words *we presumed that kids who could perform pull ups would not be overweight*, and that kids who were overweight would be unable to perform pull ups. Obesity and the ability to perform pull ups then were presumed to be mutually exclusive and not found in the same child.

Presumption # 3: The Ability To Perform Pull Ups Discourages Obesity, Encourages Self Esteem

Now if the first two presumptions were correct, we also presumed that we could decrease the odds of children being obese and having poor self esteem, by teaching them to perform pull ups. In other words as children learn to perform pull ups, their odds of being obese go down, while self esteem levels naturally go up. It's a two for one strategy. Not only that, but as self esteem and confidence go up, performance in almost every other aspect of the child's life increases. So the program multiplies itself many times over in a child's lifelong success patterns. Win/Win is certainly understating the effects of Operation PYOW.

Presumption # 4: We Can Affordably Teach Pull Ups

The final presumption we made was that we could systematically and safely teach most kids to perform pull ups by using an inexpensive height adjustable pull up bar, and a technique called leg assisted pull ups (a.k.a. Jefferson School Jump Chins). The logic of the program rolls out this way. Start 'em young, before they have a chance to pick up much excess weight, and teach kids to perform and to maintain the ability to do pull ups. With that experience in hand you've effectively vaccinated and immunized kids against ever becoming obese. Pull ups are a natural and functional antidote for obesity.

Successful? Let Me Count The Ways

Now as the result of those four years spent overseeing Operation PYOW, I can tell you that the program was successful in almost every conceivable way. For starters, the equipment and technique we used were cheap and they worked. In other words, *we taught hundreds of children to move from Wall B to Wall A in a safe, predictable, and systematic fashion without forcing anyone to participate.*

A Privilege Not An Obligation

As a matter of fact, success was introduced to each child on the first day and it continued throughout the entire program. Furthermore the whole thing was presented, in the regular classroom, as a special privilege that was earned by virtue of doing your work and behaving yourself. And when students didn't tend to the basics they lost their chance to participate in PYOW.   In short, the kids loved doing pull ups, and I doubt that there's ever been another American school who could honestly make that claim.

Parental Volunteers

The nuts and bolts of the program were tended to by parental volunteers who came in twice a week to put their class through their PYOW paces. Interestingly enough, without ever planning for it, PYOW became the primary parental involvement vehicle for the grant and the school, generating about 1500 hours of volunteer time per school year. Oh, and by the way, the parents loved it as much as the kids did. As a matter of fact several teachers felt that the parents got as much or more than the kids out of their participation.

The Private Sector

The private sector also took an interest in the program and pitched in variously to buy special PYOW Club T-shirts for the kids at the end of the school year, and donated "in kind" prizes for a "pull up a thon" fund raiser for a local charity. One year we even registered voters at a local grocery store by offering to do ten pull ups for each person who registered to vote at our booth.

And The Media Too

And the media loved the program as well writing well over two dozen complimentary articles, and covering our activities on radio and television as well. This media attention helped to solidify the program in the eyes of the kids who loved to see themselves, their friends, and their school in the paper or on the television. Realistically the media is always looking for positive things to say about kids and education, and the red, white and blue characteristics of PYOW certainly attracted their interest.

Then It Failed

Then in 1995 PYOW failed due to the lack of state funding. Actually my greatest disappointment with the program was the fact that the school, the teachers, and the neighborhood needed no grant (and nobody's permission) to continue the program. But when the grant funds dried up and went away, the program dried up and went away with it, never to be actively resurrected again.

Ten Years Later

Now, ten years later, every time I pick up a newspaper or turn on the TV somebody is talking about this nation's epidemic in childhood obesity. If it weren't for the war in Iraq I suspect it would be the number one story in the media today. And I know that multi millions are being spent on research to resolve this multi billion dollar problem, with little to no success to date.

What Every Gym Teacher Already Knows

And now I sit here knowing that every gym teacher in the nation has observed exactly what I have observed with regard to pull ups and obesity. They all know first hand that obese kids can't do pull ups, and that kids who can do pull ups can't be obese. In fact you don't have to be a teacher to be aware of that fact, just think back to your own days in gym class and you'll know exactly what I'm talking about here. You'll know intuitively that we can resolve the problem naturally and systematically by teaching kids to do pull ups...if we only choose to do so. Carpe Diem.

An Old Coach Offers a Simple Solution to Childhood Obesity

Obesity is a huge and growing problem in America and around the world. And the childhood edition of this problem is a 21st century tragedy that's not only costing our nation billions of dollars, but it's costing millions of kids their confidence, their self esteem, their willingness to try something new in public for fear of failure, and consequently their capacity to live full and productive lives.

While scientists are busy studying body chemistry, body composition, nutrition, and exercise physiology, pharmaceutical companies are busy developing more weight loss pill, the diet industry is designing a new strategies, infomercials are crowing about new exercise devices, health clubs are hustling fitness, insurance companies are cutting benefits, and McDonald's is pushing salads, all in an effort to participate in the multi billion dollar obesity industry. In the mean time, the problem continues to grow unabated, like a forest fire raging out of control.

An Old Coach's Reaction

In light of that raging forest fire I'd like to introduce you to the wisdom of a retired coach who I've known for over three decades. In the words of this old coach (he prefers to remain anonymous, and back in the shadows), "I taught physical education for most of my adult life and during that time I made the following observation. *I noticed that kids who could perform pull-ups were never obese,*" he said. "*And kids who were obese could never perform pull-ups. Pull-ups and obesity are mutually exclusive, and are never found in the same kids,*" he added.

Without Pills, Shots, or Magic Diets

The old coach's conclusion was that if you start 'em young, before they've had a chance to pick up much weight, teach them the ability to perform pull-ups, and teach them to never lose that ability, *you can immunize kids against obesity for a lifetime*, without pills, shots, magic diets, or much in the way of expense. "The more kids you can teach to physically pull their own weight," he said, "the closer you'll come to whipping the childhood obesity epidemic."

But Kids Hate Pull-Ups

I told the coach that I thought his logic was impeccable, but in my view he had one problem. According to my recollection, most kids hated pull-ups with a passion. And if they hate doing it, how can you teach them to perform pull-ups? They'll drag their feet all the way to the gym, won't they?

Using A Height Adjustable Pull-Up Bar

"Kids hate doing anything where they fail in public," the coach replied. "The trick is to start them young before they learned to fail on the pull-up bar. Start them out on a *height adjustable bar* that allows them all to succeed immediately with leg- assisted pull-ups, jumping and pulling at the same time. With this inexpensive tool you'll eliminate failure, and build regular success into the experience for all participants."

How High Do You Set The Bar

A couple of more questions popped into my mind immediately. First, how high do you set the bar when you're starting a youngster out? And secondly, how do you adjust the level of difficulty in order to insure progress? I could tell however, the wise old coach had an answer on the tip of his tongue.

The Progression

"You start the bar out low enough that the child can do at least 8 leg assisted pull-ups, but no more than 12. You allow them to work out twice a week and expect them to improve every time for a number of weeks, consecutively. In other words, in the second workout they should do 9, in the third 10, in the fourth 11, and in the fifth 12 leg assisted pull-ups. When they hit 12 repetitions you raise the bar one inch and they begin the 8-12 process all over again. This strategy allows a child to make a little progress every time he or she works out, and after several weeks they learn to EXPECT TO SUCCEED IN PUBLIC, which in turn teaches them to love instead of hate pull-ups."

They've Immunized Themselves Naturally

So if I understand it right Coach, the kids literally inch their way upward until they eventually run out of leg assistance, at which point they've not only learned to perform pull-ups, but they've also learned to love doing them, and in the process they've *immunized themselves naturally against obesity for a lifetime* as long as they maintain the ability. Does that sound about right, I asked?

They May Want To Be Bad, But...

"Mechanically speaking that's correct," the coach said. But there are a few other things that go into the strategy that you need to understand. One thing is that you're tapping into a child's natural desire to be strong and not weak. In my years of teaching *I met lots of kids who wanted to be bad, but I never met a kid who wants to be weak*. And that goes for the boys as well as the girls. We all want to be strong. All kids know that the ability to do pull-ups requires you to be strong. And when you work in a group, they're getting stronger in public, and kids love to succeed in public," he said. "They inevitably finish off by giving each other high fives, and they love every second of it."

I asked the coach what other things are built into his strategy. He said kids learn that three things make them strong, including regular work, good eating habits, and getting enough rest at night and in between workouts. They also learn that fooling around with *tobacco, alcohol, and drugs makes them weak*. And no kid ever wants to be weak. "They also learn these concepts in a very hands-on, and concrete way," he said.

Taking Responsibility For Yourself

I knew the coach could have talked on this subject all day but I wanted to finish on one other related point. The phrase *pull your own weight* has responsibility taking connotations that are very appealing to most people these days. What role does taking responsibility for oneself play in this childhood obesity prevention strategy?

After congratulating me on all the good questions the old coach said, "One of the big lessons that kids learn from working on the pull-up bar is that *nobody else can do it for you,*" he said. "I mean in reading, writing, and arithmetic you may get away with having somebody else do your homework for awhile. But the pull-up bar knows immediately if you've done the work, it knows if you're eating right, it knows if you got enough rest recently, and it pays you for doing these things with additional success. On the other hand, it also knows if you fail to do these things, and it can just as easily deny the public success that all kids crave. So this strategy absolutely encourages kids to take responsibility for themselves in all kinds of ways," the coach said.

A Web Site Dedicated to The Old Coach's Strategy

I confessed that he'd sold me. I agreed that teaching kids to pull their own weight would go a long ways towards solving the childhood obesity epidemic, it could save our nation billions of dollars, and do all kinds of wonderful things for the individuals who learned the lessons that are built into this simple, practical, affordable, and infinitely measurable strategy. In fact I was so impressed that I offered to build an informational web site dedicated to the old coach's naturalistic vision. He took me up on the offer, and as I write this sentence you can now check out www.pullyourownweight.net if you'd like to learn more about the old coach's simple childhood obesity prevention strategy.

One Final Question

My final question to parents and educators (or anyone who works with kids) is, why wait for the experts to come up with a high tech solution when you can turn the tide naturally with your own kids right now by simply teaching them to pull their own weight? As they always say, there's no time like the present. Carpe diem.

Of Height Adjustable Pull Up Bars, Leg Assisted Pull Ups, and Obesity Prevention!

"So Mr. Osbourne," Jim C. challenged in his email, "I read your article on childhood obesity prevention in the August issue of *Chicago Health and Wellness Magazine*, and I agreed when you said that kids who can do pull ups can't be overweight. I also agreed that kids who are overweight can't do pull ups, and that teaching kids how to do pull ups would do amazing things for preventing childhood obesity nationwide.

But I Disagree…

"Where I disagree with you though," Jim said, "is when you implied that pull ups are only for kids. My bet is that the strategy applies just as much to adults as to kids. That being the case, I've decided my new fitness goal to learn how to do pull ups, and to maintain that ability until the day I keel over. So I need you to explain the height adjustable pull up bar concept, and the leg assisted pull ups in a little more detail, including where can I get a height adjustable pull up bar? I've never seen one before."

The World's Simplest Wellness Program

Well Jim, if I implied that pull ups were only for kids, let me offer you my sincerest apologies. You're of course 100% right when you say this strategy applies to anyone, at any age. Also, I applaud your new goal. It'll serve you well for years to come. And since you're an adult, you can label it the world's simplest wellness program.

The Height Adjustable Pull Up Bar

Now then, a height adjustable pull up bar is exactly what it says...a pull up bar whose height is adjustable higher or lower, ideally in one inch increments. In fact it should be adjustable from a location right below your chin when your feet are flat on the floor, to a location where the bar is well above your head in a position where your arms are fully extended, with no bend in your elbows.

The Eight to Twelve Rule

If you have one of these units in hand, the strategy is to experiment a little in order to determine the bar height at which you can do *at least eight repetitions* of leg assisted pull ups (jumping and pulling at the same time) but *no more than twelve*. In workout number one, I suggest you do eight leg assisted pull ups (LAPU's), and you may want to repeat this one or two times (i.e. two to three sets) per workout. In workout number two you will do nine LAPU's, in workout number three ten, in number four eleven, and in workout number five you'll do twelve LAPU's. Congrats!

Raising the Bar, One Inch at a Time

Now when you hit twelve repetitions, that's an indication that you should *raise the bar one inch* and begin the entire eight to twelve repetition scenario all over again. The idea here is to safely create *very thin layers of improvement* workout after workout, week after week, month after month until the bar is so high that you've run out of leg assistance. At that point you will have the ability to do real live pull ups, and you'll be unable to carry much excess baggage when you get there. But don't surprised if this process takes several months to complete…but it's well worth it, I promise.

Getting Enough Rest

A couple other things need to be added here, including the fact that you should plan to do *minimally two, and maximally three workouts per week* on non-consecutive days of the week. This will allow your body to recover from workout to workout, and you will continue to make enviable progress for weeks on end, which will stoke your motivation and inspire you to follow all the way through to the end, because you've learned how to approach this daunting task like eating an elephant, one bite at a time.

Eat Right, and Avoid Tobacco, Alcohol, and Drugs

Another thing, regular progress will also depend heavily on your ability to clean up bad eating habits, because the pull up bar pays you to be both strong and light. Simply put, the stronger and lighter you are, the more pull ups you'll be able to do. The bar also pays you to steer clear of tobacco, alcohol, and drugs, *all of which inevitably render you weaker, not stronger.* Again, you're no different than the kids in this respect.

In other words, regular work, together with good eating habits, sufficient rest, and avoiding the negative habits of tobacco, alcohol, and drugs will make you a little bit stronger every week, every month, every quarter, etc until at the end, those slices pile up and you'll be stronger in all kinds of ways, including on the pull up bar.

Try Googling Height Adjustable Pull Up Bars

With regard to where you can purchase a height adjustable pull up bar, I can only say that this is a fitness column, not an ad for any specific piece of equipment. But if you were to sit down at your computer and Google "height adjustable pull up bars," my bet is that you'd come up with all kinds of valuable information.

At worst, I've seen people build height adjustable bars from parts (pipe and one inch chain) purchased at their local hardware store. After all, we're not talking about anything complicated or expensive here. And once you've successfully mastered the ability to do pull ups, you can use the closest tree limb for your workout, kind of like Tom and Huck, or Godzilla the Gorilla. One final note, this strategy was originally developed by, and is fully approved by Mother Nature herself. Banana anyone?

Every Body's Different, Every Body Can Make Regular Progress, And Regular Progress IS Winning!

Presuming you have more than one child in the program, one of the things kids learn in *Operation Pull Your Own Weight (OPYOW)* is that *every body is different*. And I do mean every body. Some bodies are tall while others are short. Some bodies are light while others are heavy. Some bodies are male, while others are female. Bodies even come in a multitude, a veritable rainbow of different colors, and each one is unique and different from the other, which is why the pull-up bar in this program is height adjustable...to accommodate all these different kinds of bodies.

Every Body Can Get Stronger

On the other hand, another thing kids learn in OPYOW is that if you accommodate all these different kinds of bodies, *every body can make regular progress* towards the goal of being able to Pull Your Own Weight, towards getting strong, and towards immunizing yourself against obesity for a lifetime. And when I say regular progress I mean that...done right, **every time** a kid grabs onto the pull-up bar, he or she will be better, stronger, and closer to becoming immunized against obesity than the last time. And this predictable progress will continue for a good six to eight weeks.

Collective Success Is Built In

Done right, **every kid** learns to *expect improvement*, **every kid** expects to be stronger, **every kid** expects that **all the other kids** will improve **every time** they have the opportunity to work out on the pull-up bar. And after each successful set of pull-ups, kids give each other high fives, and revel in one another's success. Done right, this *collective expectation of success **is built into** Operation Pull Your Own Weight.*

Regular Improvement = Winning

Another thing kids learn in OPYOW is that *regular improvement **is winning**, and that **winning is improving**, getting stronger on a regular basis.* They also learn that getting stronger on a regular basis requires regular work, good eating habits, sufficient rest, and avoiding negative habits like tobacco, alcohol, and drugs. As a matter of fact they also learn the reverse, namely that without regular workouts, good eating habits, sufficient rest, and without avoiding tobacco, alcohol, and drugs, you are choosing to be weak. And as we've said on previous occasions, NO KID WANTS TO BE WEAK!

Done Right, Every Body's A Winner

When presented right, you have kids standing in line at the annual fall fest, twelve and fifteen deep, all night long, *paying money for the opportunity* to get on the pull up bar and show their parents how strong they're becoming. You have fifty-out-of-fifty kids who actively choose pull-ups over recess. And in one case, you have an entire (at-risk) school full of kids who take pride in their ability to Pull Their Own Weight. In other words, when presented right, in OPYOW, there are NO LOSERS, NO FAILURES. THERE ARE ONLY WINNERS. So make sure and present it right.

P.S. On the pull-up bar *these lessons are learned in a very concrete (non-abstract, non-theoretical) way.* In other words it's not just more talk, it's real live, hands-on, interactive action that gets built into PYOW participants at a very practical level.

Privilege VS Obligation In Learning To Pull Your Own Weight

As he reached the last rung on the monkey bars, his face grimacing, his little hands grabbing hold and hanging on tight, Billy Jr. dropped to the ground, beamed with pride, and crowed, "Dad, did you see that? I made it all the way to the end!"

Bill Sr. smiled broadly at his son and gave him a high five. "You're really getting strong aren't you Billy," his dad said with a tangible sense of pride in his own voice.

Kids Naturally Revel In Physical Achievement

Now with this picture in mind, you'll know what I mean when I say that *kids naturally enjoy, even revel in their physical achievements* starting with the first finger they grab, and the first step they take. And just because a task is difficult and challenging doesn't mean that it's any less enjoyable for kids. As long as the goal is valued, (i.e. reaching the last rung on the monkey bars) difficulty even increases the enjoyment.

Kids Are Naturally Curious and Creative

Kids are not naturally lazy and slothful. On the contrary, they're natural born explorers of their environments. They're curious about everything and everyone around them. When they see it, they naturally want to reach out and touch it, grab it, taste it, smell it, hear it, and experience it as fully as possible. That's how and why kids grow so quickly in their formative years.

Privilege VS Obligation

Since kids are naturally programmed to explore themselves and the world around them, *the challenge for a legitimate educator* is to tap into that natural curiosity, to cultivate it, to encourage it, to grow it, day after day, week after week, month after month. But in order for that to happen, education must be presented and perceived as something the child gets to do, not something the child has to do. In other words, education must be seen as a privilege, an opportunity, instead of an obligation, a job.

Keeping The Flame Lit...

When this challenge is met, and this goal is achieved, the child's natural sense of curiosity will remain inflamed, and they will continue to soak in new knowledge from new experiences, and they will also come to understand and appreciate the fulfillment that learning, in the best sense, has to offer.

Or Extinguishing It

On the contrary, when we inadvertently turn education into a job, complete with commutes, daily starting times, tasks that have to be completed whether the child wants to do them or not, and extrinsic rewards (i.e. stars and grades) that transform the natural born learner into an object to be compared and judged against others, the flame is extinguished. The child quickly learns that what adults call education is not fun, is not something you get to do, is not a privilege, but a job, an obligation, and something to avoid whenever possible. Kids and teachers live for the weekend, and summer vacation.

Regular Improvement Feeds The Flame

For these reasons, it's essential for anyone wanting to teach a child to physically *Pull Their Own Weight*, that pull-ups be presented and perceived as something the child gets to do, not something they have to do. And the key to growing that curiosity flame and that privileged status lies in making sure the child walks away from each experience feeling successful, feeling better this time than last time, feeling as if there was a payoff for the time and effort invested. We'll explore that topic next.

Bad But Not Weak...

Until next time remember, lots of kids today want to be bad. But you'll never meet a kid who wants to be weak. They all want to be strong.

"Some Kids Want To Be Bad, But No Kids Want To Be Weak"

One of the important strategies of *Operation Pull Your Own Weight* is to **exchange the terms** good and bad, for the terms strong and weak in your child's vocabulary. Why you ask? In the seventeen years I spent teaching and coaching, I met plenty of kids who "wanted to be bad." But I never met one who "wanted to be weak."

Girls, Boys, All Ages...

That goes for girls as well as boys, regardless of age, race, ethnicity, religion, etc. Think about for a second, have you ever known anyone who actually wanted to be weak? Personally I've never known anyone, who ever knew anyone, who actually wanted to be weak. We all want to be strong. It's just how human beings are programmed. And for most kids, being able to perform pull-ups is a sure sign of physical strength.

What Does It Take?

But what does it take to develop strength on the pull-up bar? According to the OPYOW recipe it takes...

- regular work (twice per week),
- eating right,
- getting enough rest,
- and avoiding tobacco, alcohol and drugs.

In other words we taught kids that if they worked out on the pull-up bar a couple times each week, ate right, got sufficient rest, and avoided tobacco, alcohol, and drugs, they'd get stronger on the pull-up bar. We also taught kids that if they failed to work out regularly, if they ate poorly, failed to get enough rest, and messed with tobacco, alcohol, and drugs, they were shooting themselves in the foot, and asking to be weak.

No Way! That'll Make Me Weak!!!

In fact I had a kindergartner back in the Jefferson School days who, in front a class full of kids, looked up at me and said, "Coach, my uncle Freddie wanted me to smoke a cigarette with him last night, but I told him, "No way. That'll make me weak." I immediately gave this youngster five, as did his teacher, and the rest of his classmates who all understood that messing with tobacco, alcohol, and drugs make you weak! And as we said previously, none of these kids wanted to be weak in anything.

Readin', Writin', and Rithmatic Too.....

Interestingly enough, those same kids who want to avoid weakness on the pull-up bar, also want to avoid weakness in all other aspects of their lives too, including their academics. And interestingly enough the habits that make you strong on the pull-up bar are the exact same habits that make you strong in every other aspect of life as well. If you work at reading (writin' or rithmatic) regularly, over a period of time, eat right, get plenty of rest, and avoid negative habits like tobacco, alcohol, and drugs, you'll eventually be strong in reading (writin' and rithmatic), taking it one step at a time.

In Conclusion...

In conclusion, done correctly, the lessons you teach on the pull-up bar carry over to all other aspects of a child's life because, as we've said a number of times now, some of them may want to be bad, but none of them ever want to be weak. If you make your case in these terms, your kids understand, they'll respond positively, and they will develop *not only physical strength, but an inner strength and confidence* (self esteem) in themselves and their ability to meet challenges, and to overcome obstacles. Is there a better lesson you can teach a child at a young age? Personally, I can't think of one.

Nobody Else Can Do It For You

We've suggested so far that *Operation Pull Your Own Weight* must be presented and perceived as an opportunity, a privilege instead of an obligation or a job. And to be perceived that way, it helps to make OPYOW a social affair, and to take advantage of the collective expectations of success that can be cultivated in the social setting. You should also tap into every child's burning desire to become strong and avoid weakness, and all these are important stage setters for the next point we'd like to make.

It's Automatically Built In

An automatic, built in lesson for OPYOW participants is the realization that *nobody else can Pull Your Own Weight for you.* Only you can take the responsibility for doing that. In other words, nobody else can do the work for you. Nobody else can eat the right foods for you. Nobody else can get enough rest for you. And nobody can avoid tobacco, alcohol, and drugs for you. If you don't do these things for yourself, you'll lose the opportunity to become stronger every week, every month, etc., and you'll be inadvertently choosing to become weak.

You Can't Cheat the Pull Up Bar

In an age when copying a friend's homework is commonplace, even acceptable as long as you don't get caught, **YOU CANNOT CHEAT THE PULL UP BAR!** If you fail to fit the workouts in, if you fail to control your eating and sleeping habits, and if you dabble in tobacco, alcohol, and drugs, the pull-up bar will tell you immediately, and in no uncertain terms, by denying you the progress you expect to make each time you grab onto the bar. You may even get weaker. In short, the pull-up bar pulls no punches.

Of Pull-Ups and Homework

And interestingly enough, like the other concepts we've talked about so far, the rules that apply to the pull-up bar, also apply to all the other aspects of a child's life, including their academic achievements. That is to say, you may get away with cheating on your homework in the short term. But in the long run, if you want to get strong in readin', writin', and arithmetic, nobody else can do the work for you. You have to do it yourself...just exactly like the pull-up bar. You must take responsibility for the various kinds of strength that you develop, and do the things

64

necessary to earn them. In the end your life is your life and nobody else can live it for you. The ball is indeed in your court.

Childhood Obesity and Personal Responsibility Taking Behavior

The Robert Woods Johnson Foundation recently announced that it's contributing $500 Million Dollars over the next five years to combat the growing crisis in childhood obesity. The RWJF expects to work with the Feds, state governments, and schools who have already spent billions trying to turn the tide on this problem. Celebrities are speaking up, business leaders getting involved, and I just read where a tri-athlete has dedicated his next event to "raising public awareness of childhood."

But at this point I need to raise my hand and ask, how much more money are we going to throw at this problem without making the slightest dentin it? How much more aware can we get? If it weren't for the war in Iraq, childhood obesity would be the number one issue in the news today.

Personal Responsibility Taking Behavior

Sooner or later someone needs to point out an obvious flaw in the midst of all this mega spending, out speaking, and awareness raising. Someone besides

McDonald's needs to recognize that we can spend money until we're blue in the face, we can speak out, and market the bejeebers out of the conventional "eat right and exercise more" anti obesity message. But until we address the lack of personal responsibility taking behavior that lies at the bottom of this problem, we'll continue spinning our wheels, wasting time and money to beat the childhood obesity problem. In order to succeed, something must change.

It's Preventable, But Only If…

We need to recognize that Childhood obesity is a PREVENTABLE PROBLEM, but only if victims learn to take responsibility for what goes in their mouths, and how many calories they burn each day. Kids must learn to avoid junk food, TV, and video games, just like they must learn to avoid tobacco, alcohol, and drugs.

But How Can We Do It?

So how, you may ask, can we systematically teach our kids to eat right, get sufficient rest, plenty of exercise, and to avoid tobacco alcohol and drugs? How do we teach our kids to TAKE RESPONSIBILITY FOR THEIR OWN LIVES when everything around them encourages kids to DEPEND ON governments and business for the goods and services from which THEY (governments and businesses) PROFIT?

There are probably other good answers to this troublesome question, but I'm only familiar with one. It's called Operation Pull Your Own Weight. It's incredibly simple, incredibly inexpensive, and I watched it work with elementary school kids for four consecutive years (1990-1994) at Jefferson Elementary School in Davenport, IA. With that intro, here are the basic principals for Operation Pull Your Own Weight along with the ways in which it specifically addresses childhood obesity.

The Basic Premise

The basic underlying premise of OPYOW is that kids who can do pull ups can't carry much excess body weight, and kids who carry much excess body weight can't do pull ups. So the idea is to develop our kid's ability to do pull ups, and then encourage them to maintain that ability right on through adulthood. To accomplish this simple feat is to naturally immunize kids against obesity for a lifetime.

How Can We Do That?

If you accept this basic premise, the next question becomes, how do you teach kids to do pull ups, when pull ups are the most universally hated exercise on the planet?

You have to start by recognizing that it's not really pull ups that kids hate. It's FAILING IN FRONT OF THEIR PEERS that kids hate.

Kids who can do pull ups and who succeed in front of their peers, don't hate pull ups. In fact they enjoy being able to tackle a difficult task like pull ups, and succeed in front of their peers. It becomes a badge of honor, a status symbol. I personally witnessed an entire school full of kids learning to love pull ups back in the early nineties.

Here's the Key

So then, how do you make pull ups accessible to all kids, and transform hated failure into joyful success? You use a simple device called a HEIGHT ADJUSTABLE PULL UP BAR (it raises and lowers in one inch increments) in conjunction with LEG ASSISTED PULL UPS (encouraging kids to jump and pull simultaneously) which allows almost all kids to succeed on the pull up bar immediately in front of their peers, week after week after week. Because of their continual success, participants look forward to the opportunity to tackle a difficult task and to succeed front of their peers. At that point pull ups become valued instead of despised. Let me explain.

The Starting Point

The idea is to allow kids to keep their feet on the ground, lower the bar to a point where they can jump and pull simultaneously, and easily perform eight leg assisted pull ups in workout number one. In workout # 2 the children are allowed to do nine pull ups. In workout # 3 they're allowed to do ten, in # 4 eleven, and finally in workout # 5 they're allowed to do twelve pull ups.

Once they develop the ability to do 12 pull ups at one level, the bar is raised ONE INCH and the whole eight to twelve routine is repeated over and over again until their pull up goal (the ability to do one real pull up) is reached. Sometimes it takes several months for kids to eventually run out of leg assistance and to reach the point where they're finally doing real live pull ups...IN FRONT OF THEIR PEERS and loving every second of it.

In the wake of each and every workout every child is instantly congratulated by their peers and their teacher, thus kids learn to succeed and to feel good about themselves every time their hands hit the pull up bar! Kids automatically develop physical confidence in themselves under these conditions.

An Opportunity Not an Obligation

At Jefferson Elementary School, pull ups were always treated as an opportunity (you got to do pull ups) not an obligation (you had to do pull ups). Kids were "allowed" to work out only twice a week, and to do only one pull up more than they did last time.

Strong VS Weak, Not Good VS Bad

OPYOW also took full advantage of every kid's desire to be strong and to avoid being weak…at anything. Have you ever met a child who wants to be weak at anything? And the ability to do pull ups is universally associated with being strong. In other words we never talked about avoiding obesity. We always talked about getting stronger on the pull up bar. The conversation was always positive, and we avoided negativity.

Lessons Bred Into OPYOW Participants

And how does a kid grow strong on the pull up bar? There are six simple answers to this question and teachers were constantly reinforcing them throughout the PYOW experience. In a very hands-on way kids learned that, in order to gain strength on the pull up bar they had to work regularly, eat right, get sufficient rest at night, and they had to avoid using tobacco, alcohol, and drugs.

On the flip side they learned that if they failed to do the work, if they ate much junk food, if they didn't get enough rest, and if they fooled around with tobacco, alcohol and drugs, they'd be making themselves weak not strong. And as we said before, there's no such thing as a kid who wants to be weak at anything.

This point cannot be overstated so I'll repeat it once more. These kids were exposed week after week after week to the lessons of OPYOW which included…

•   Gaining strength (on the bar) is an opportunity not a right – in other words, in this school you could be denied the opportunity to get on pull up bar if you failed to get your work done or you misbehaved in class…a reward for good behavior.

•   You gain strength through regular work

•   You gain strength by eating right

•   You gain strength by getting enough rest

•   You become weak by fooling around with tobacco, alcohol, and drugs

•   Kids also learned that NOBODY CAN DO IT FOR THEM

- Kids learned to tackle a difficult task and to succeed in public by setting concrete goals, and growing in small, but regular, predictable increments.
- In other words, as the result of learning to perform pull ups, KIDS LEARNED PERSONAL RESPONSIBILITY TAKING BEHAVIORS.

Self Respect, Self Confidence, and Dignity

Interestingly enough the same principles that apply to strength gain on the pull up bar also apply to strength gain in reading, writing, arithmetic, and anything else in life. And by participating in OPYOW, kids not only immunize themselves against obesity for a lifetime, but they also develop a tangible sense of self respect, self confidence, and dignity that are cultivated most effectively when the PYOW seed is planted at a young age, and allowed to develop right on into adulthood.

Systematic Repercussions Not Forgotten...

None of the previous commentary is intended to negate the role that the system plays in aggravating problems like childhood obesity. That's blatant, obvious, and it needs to be addressed.

But to the degree that kids learn to take responsibility for their own lives, in as many ways as possible, they'll grow strong, despite the system. To the degree they fail to take responsibility, they'll be victimized by the system. And in the end, only strong people are capable of tackling difficult tasks like improving a problematic system. So hats off to those kids who learn to pull their own weight at a young age, and who master themselves instead of becoming mastered by the system. They're the hope of the world.

Embarrassed When Communicating With Your Kids Over Childhood Obesity?

A 10 Point Strategy To Make The Experience Positive

With childhood obesity growing exponentially, like a forest fire raging out of control, one big challenge for parents and teachers is to find ways to communicate with kids about the problem *without offending or embarrassing them*. After all, if you're unable to communicate, how can you resolve the problem? In light of that challenge, here are ten things to keep in mind when communicating with your kids on obesity.

1. *Start young*, before they have a chance to pick up too much excess weight. As a matter of fact, the younger you start, the better the odds become of avoiding childhood obesity, which almost inevitably turns into adult obesity.

2. *Avoid negative terms* like fat, obese, and chubby unless you want to offend the youngster's self perception, and all that goes along with it. That's a

75

dead end street, with no redeeming qualities, and you should avoid it completely.

3. Instead, couch your conversations in terms of *how to get stronger and avoid weakness.* In many years of school teaching I met lots of kids who wanted to be bad, but I never met a kid (boy or girl) who wanted to be weak in anything (and that includes reading, writing, and arithmetic). Weakness in your kid's world is UNCOOL. However, BAD is just another way of saying strong, resilient, and uncompromising. So in place of good and bad, substitute strong and weak.

4. *Choose an activity that pays for a child to get both stronger and lighter*, and then teach them how to improve, in public, on a regular basis, over a period of time. Done correctly the child's public success, and the praise that follows, will show them that they can try new things in public (they can take a risk) without embarrassing themselves, feeling ostracized or alienated by failure. Done right this activity will strengthen self-perception instead of undermine it.

5. This activity could take a variety of forms, *but the simplest example is pull ups*. I suggest pull ups for several reasons, starting with the fact that they're simple, everyone understands them, they require little space, and almost no money. Also most kids usually associate pull ups with being strong.

6. And as any gym teacher will gladly confirm, kids who can do pull ups are never obese. And kids who are obese can never do pull ups. In other words, developing a kid's ability to do pull ups, along with his/her desire to maintain it, *immunizes them against obesity for a lifetime, naturally, without pills, shots, or special diets.*

7. Using a *height adjustable bar* along with a technique called *leg assisted pull ups*, where a child jumps and pulls at the same time, *allows all kids to experience immediate and continued success*. And by inching the bar higher and higher, they eventually run out of leg assistance and they're doing real live pull ups.

8. Always treat pull ups as *an opportunity instead of an obligation*. That is to say this activity should be something your kids get to do (like Disneyland)

instead of something they have to do (like clean their room). It should be a reward not a job. Done right, you can use the opportunity to do pull ups as the reward for cleaning their room. Until the room is clean Johnny, we'll do no pull ups and you'll miss out on the opportunity to get stronger.

9. *Lessons packed between the lines of this strategy include* the fact that regular work, good eating habits, and getting sufficient rest (at night and in between workouts) MAKES A PARTICIPANT STRONG. On the other hand, the lack of regular work, poor eating and rest habits, along with counterproductive behaviors such as using tobacco, alcohol, and drugs MAKES A PARTICIPANT WEAK. And again, *I've never met a child who wants to be weak in anything.* Have you?

10. The other hands-on lesson that you can teach is *personal responsibility.* In other words if someone else does your homework on the pull up bar, you make no gains. Nobody else can do the work for you...it's totally up to you.

Now, if this strategy has you intrigued sufficiently, you can learn lots more by checking the web site www.pullyourownweight.com. As a matter of fact, among other things you'll find a stage setting story called "*A Really Strong Story For Kids*" that you can print off and read to your own kids so that they have a good solid understanding of the strength building strategy you're about to implement. Done right, *you can immunize your kids against obesity for a lifetime without ever resorting to pills, shots, or special diets*. And if you've read this far you already know… the rest is up to you.

P.S. What if you've failed to start 'em young before they've had a chance to pick up much excess weight? What if they're in junior high, high school or beyond, and they're already significantly overweight and deathly scared of anything that smells like a pull up bar? What then?

My suggestion is that *the golden rule of pull ups is equally true for kids from three to ninety three*. That is to say if you can do pull ups you can't carry much excess weight, and if you carry much excess weight you can't do pull ups.

However, almost anyone at any age can use a height adjustable bar together with leg assisted pull ups to generate immediate access/success. Furthermore, almost anyone can inch the bar higher and higher over time, combining regular workouts with improved eating and rest habits, and produce thin slices of improvement over weeks and months until they can physically pull their own weight. And when they reach their goal, they've immunized themselves against obesity for a lifetime without pills, shots, or special diets, as long as they never lose that hard won ability. It's about that simple.

Thin, But Regular Slices of Improvement, the Key to Motivating Kids, and Preventing Childhood Obesity

The journey of a thousand miles starts with a single step. And how do you eat an elephant? You do it one step at a time, of course. But when working with young kids (K-3) developing their ability to do pull ups and to immunize themselves against obesity, we always talked in terms of stacking thin slices of improvement on top of each other week after week, month after month, until in the long run, THEY ADDED UP TO A WHOLE PILE OF SUCCESS.

The Kids Get It

The first reason I tell you this is because *the kids understood this analogy*. It always seemed to get my point across, and it's always good to know something that just plain works. I even had occasions where visually demonstrated the point with slices of Velveeta cheese, or sheets of typing paper…whatever was handy to make sure the kids understood the importance of making regular progress over time.

It Motivates Them

The second reason I tell you about the thin slices of improvement concept is that it was *the absolute KEY to motivating these kids*. In other words, the effect of succeeding just a little bit, in front of their peers, week after week, month after month was to *create positive expectations*, not only from individual participants, but from their peers who are also learning to expect the participant TO SUCCEED AGAIN AND AGAIN. Collective expectations are incredibly powerful motivators for kids and adults.

They all begin to think, "She did eight pull ups last time without too much effort. With a little more effort she'll be able to do nine this time." The same thought process turns nine pull ups into ten, and ten into eleven, and eleven into twelve, etc.

Thin Slices and Whole Piles of Success

After five successful experiences on the pull up bar, in front of their peers, the bar is raised literally one inch, and the entire eight to twelve scenario begins all over again. The child then thinks, "Wow, I did twelve at the previous level without too much effort, I can surely do eight at this new height." As the bar is raised one inch at a time, over weeks and months, the child inevitably runs out of leg assistance, and these incredibly thin but regular slices of improvement develop into the ability to do real live pull ups, which collectively constitutes a WHOLE PILE OF SUCCESS.

Confidence That Drowns Out the Fear of Failure

And when the day comes when the success fails to happen and (s)he doesn't improve, the participant still has a history of public success, which translates into positive expectations that guard him or her against the fear of public failure and humiliation. In other words, everyone, including the participant himself, knows if he keeps working at it, that success is bound to follow.

Pull Ups, Reading, Writing, and Arithmetic

This is how you teach kids to love doing pull ups. This is also how you teach kids to love reading, writing, and arithmetic. What works on the pull up bar, works in the classroom, and what works on the pull up bar, works in life. It all boils down to stacking those thin slices of success, week after week, month after month, year after year. If you can teach a child that lesson he or she will grow stronger and stronger in all kinds of ways and you will have done them the biggest favor any teacher could ever do. Amen.

Thin Slices of Progress Fuel the Motivational Flame

When it comes to the issue of childhood obesity, the BIG QUESTION is always, "How do you motivate kids to exercise more, eat less/better?" And once you have them in motion, "How do you keep them in motion?" Then to make matters even more challenging I want to answer the question, "How can *Operation Pull Your Own Weight* even hope to motivate kids by focusing on the one exercise that's almost universally hated by kids around the country?"

Progress Motivates Like Nothing Else

I'll answer that question in one word, "PROGRESS." More specifically, if the kids you're working with can make regular, predictable, quantifiable progress, in public, almost every time they grab onto the pull up bar, *they quickly learn to expect progress*. They also learn that *progress occurs in thin, but tangible slices*. They learn that when those thin slices are piled on top of one another week after week, month after month, year after year, *they add up to a whole bunch of progress*. And finally they absorb this information at a *very concrete, practical, hands-on level* when working on a pull-up bar.

They Want A Return On Their Investment

Let's say this in another way. I've observed that kids want to see a regular return on their investment of time, effort, and energy. They also want to avoid wasting their time, effort, and energy in activities that fail to yield a profit. Finally, and perhaps most importantly, they want to avoid investing any of their social capital in activities that could result in public failure and humiliation…such as being unable to do a pull-up in front of their friends. As we've said on previous occasions, there are some kids who'll tell you they want to be bad, but NO KIDS WANT TO BE WEAK AT ANYTHING.

Set The Stage Right And Win

So the trick is to start young, and set the stage in such as way that the time, effort, and energy your kids invest, yields a small, but tangible profit such as the ability to say, "Hey, I'm stronger today than the last time we did pull-ups, and I'll be even stronger next week, just wait and see." That is to say, if you set the stage right, your kids will quickly learn that regular work in conjunction with eating right, getting enough rest, and avoiding tobacco, alcohol, and drugs will make them stronger in every way (physically, mentally, socially, and spiritually). AND ALL KIDS WANT TO BE STRONG IN EVERYTHING.

It Works For Reading, Writing, And Arithmetic Too

Now that's how you light the motivational flame in Operation Pull Your Own Weight on the pull-up bar, and keep it burning for a lifetime. And by the way, the same formula works for reading, writing, and arithmetic too. Now let me end by proposing a toast to a generation of kids who learn to Pull Their Own Weight in all kinds of ways.

The Many Virtues of Infinite Measurability

One of the major stumbling blocks in defeating childhood obesity is the lack of measurability, a way to conveniently evaluate progress, which results in a lack of motivation, and an epidemic that continues to grow like a forest fire raging out of control.

As a matter of fact the National Institute of Medicine recently (9/14/05) issued a disturbing report indicating that after spending over $68,000,000 over five years on just one program (there were many others), because of poor evaluation methods, we still have no idea what works and what doesn't work. We wasted $68,000,000...surprise, surprise.

If You Can't Measure It, How Do You Know?

But if you lack the ability to measure accurately how will you ever know if you're winning, losing, or just spinning your wheels? The State of Arkansas for example, is considered to be one of the nation's leaders in the battle against childhood obesity. Bill Clinton has even gotten into the fray. They decided to measure every child's body mass index (the most commonly used indicator) and put it on their report card once every quarter...in other words, every nine weeks.

How Do You Motivate Kids

But even if this measurement is accurate and meaningful for kids, which is highly questionable in itself, getting feedback once every nine weeks packs almost no motivational punch at all. By the same token it's economically impractical to do it daily, weekly, or even monthly. Once a quarter is about the best they can do.

Other more sophisticated measurement possibilities such as measuring percentage of body fat via electronic impedance (computer) or underwater weighing are dramatically more expensive and much less likely to be used by anyone except a professor or grad student in a university physiology lab. Furthermore, their model focuses on a negative factor...how fat are you. So lacking regular feedback, in combination with its negative connotations DOOM the most common strategies to failure. And after years of work and multi millions in expenditure, we still don't know what works and what doesn't work.

A Kindergartner Can Measure This

In contrast, the measurability factor in a program called Operation Pull Your Own Weight is very regular and highly practical. You need no special instruments, no magic formulas, and almost no specialized training to tell if a student, or a group of students are improving or not. If you can count from one to twelve, as most kindergartners can do, you qualify. As a matter of fact, elementary school age kids not only can, but they have measured themselves and others without problems. Not only that but what you're focusing on in this program (strength gain) has positive not negative connotations.

The Feedback is Frequent

More specifically, using a height adjustable pull up bar and leg assisted pull ups, the idea is to count and record the number of repetitions a participant can do at a particular bar height. The basic idea is to find a bar height at which the participant can do eight leg assisted pull ups which constitutes workout # one. In workout # 2 they do nine, in workout # 3 they do ten, in workout # 4 they do eleven, and in workout # 5 they do twelve leg assisted pull ups. Then in workout # 6 the bar is raised one inch and the whole eight to twelve scenario begins all over again.

And the Motivation is High

In other words each participant is shown how to improve regularly, in very small increments every week, every month, over a prescribed period of time. The progress is highly visible, INFINITELY MEASUREABLE, and the feedback occurs every single time the participant works out.

Under these conditions, including feedback every time you work out, along with public success and celebration (high fives), motivation remains high throughout the program, evaluation becomes extremely easy and affordable, and the focus (strength gain not fat loss) is positive not negative. In other words, Operation Pull Your Own Weight is extremely affordable, extremely motivating, and INFINITELY MEASUREABLE AND EVALUATEABLE.

In the End, You'll Know

At the end of a week, a month, a quarter, a year, you'll know, unequivocally, if you're winning the war, losing the war, or just treading water. You'll never be in a position where you've spent $68,000,000 and still not know what you were trying to find out. Not only that, but you'll defeat childhood obesity naturally, without resorting to pills, shots, and special diets to get the job done. What more can you ask?

Make OPYOW
A Social Affair

Last time we talked about making pull-ups and opportunity or a privilege instead of an obligation or a job. And one way you can accomplish this goal is to make sure your PYOW sessions are social affairs in which you're coaching at least two, if not three or four kids at the same time. This arrangement makes it more fun for your kids, and it allows each of them to witness one another's continued success, giving high fives, and collectively appreciating how strong they're all becoming.

Start Off Real Easy

Now in order for this to really work, it's essential that you customize each child's workout in such a way that they're starting out at a level that's EASY for them. Remember, you want to sneak up on this thing, and get used to it, before it becomes a real challenge, which it will soon enough.

Build In Regular Success

By starting each child at an easy level, it allows you to build regular success (one more repetition, one more resistance level) into the PYOW experience. Done right, each child will improve every time they work out for at least the first six to eight weeks. This strategy *sets the PYOW stage in such a way that each child EXPECTS TO IMPROVE*, expects to get high fives and pats on the back, expects that there's a payoff for the time/effort invested, and they begin looking forward to each new PYOW experience. Now that's no small task.

We're All Getting Stronger

Under these conditions all the participants will see that everyone is getting stronger, and *they'll learn to celebrate and feel good about other kid's wins as well as their own.* They'll all see that Jimmie or Susie CAN DO IT, just like the rest of us. Collective peer appreciation and validation is *an extremely potent form of motivation.*

When you start things off in this way, and kids are expecting to get stronger and they begin to understand that regular work, good eating and resting habits do payoff. And when the inevitable challenges come (and they will), your kids will hang in there, they'll persist, and they'll overcome the hurdles that would intimidate and defeat children who lack these experiences and these expectations

We used to tell kids that laying thin slices of success/improvement on top of one another week after week, month after month, eventually yields a whole pile of success…and they understood that.

Tap Into The Power of Collective Expectations

The moral of this post is that, if you make PYOW a social affair and tap into the power of collective expectations of success, the kids will continue looking forward to the opportunity to grab hold of the pull-up bar and show the world, along with their friends, that they too can pull their own weight, that they too are getting stronger as they work regularly at it, and that they too CAN DO IT!

A Childhood Obesity Prevention Program Generates Instant and Delayed Gratification Simultaneously

Teaching kids to immunize themselves against obesity by teaching them to perform pull ups (obese kids can't do pull ups) with a height adjustable pull up bar (HAPUB) and leg assisted pull ups (LAPU's) provides instant and delayed gratification simultaneously. Check out the strategy and the childhood obesity prevention technique called *Operation Pull Your Own Weight.*

Height Adjustable Pull-Up Bars, Leg Assisted Pull Ups

Using a height adjustable pull up bar allows students to start with their feet planted firmly on the ground in order to perform leg assisted pull ups, where they're encouraged to jump and pull at the same time. The bar is placed low enough that participants can do at least eight leg assisted pull ups in their first workout, succeeding right away in front of their peers, creating immediate gratification.

Learning to Love Pull Ups

In workout number two *they're allowed* to do nine, in workout number three they do ten, in workout number four they do eleven, and in workout number five they do twelve leg assisted pull ups. When they can do twelve LAPU's, the bar is *raised one full inch*, and the entire eight to twelve repetition scenario is repeated all over again. Done correctly most participants will improve just a little bit, every time they workout for eight or ten weeks straight, and in the process they lose their fear of the pull up bar and actually learn to look forward to their opportunity to perform successfully, in public.

Instant Combined With Delayed Gratification

By using the height adjustable pull up bar together with leg assisted pull ups, students can literally "inch their way up towards the ultimate goal of doing real live, conventional pull ups. The long-term goal of being able to do pull ups often takes weeks, months, or even a year to complete. *This translates into delayed gratification.*

But on the way to reaching that ultimate goal, the regular, but thin slices of success provide the immediate gratification, fan the motivational flame, and teaches participants to "expect success" (confidence/self esteem) not failure. It also teaches them to persist, persist, and persist in order to achieve that ultimate goal that they've set for themselves.

It Works With the Three R's Too

Interestingly enough the "thin slices of success strategy," with its built in instant and delayed gratifications, works not only for pull ups, but for reading, writing, and arithmetic too. Educators who successfully teach kids to understand their experience on the pull up bar, can easily *translate that experience into the academic arena*. In the process they'll cultivate self confident and highly motivated kids who can handle delayed gratification and immunize themselves against obesity at the same time, as long as they maintain the ability to do pull ups.

Great Expectations

Your self esteem sets a stage for your <u>expectations</u> of the world and how you interact with it. If you really can see yourself as strong, physically capable, intelligent, confident, (not cocky) yet sensitive to, and respectful of other people, you'll <u>expect</u> other people to see you in the same light. It will reflect in the way you carry yourself; walking, talking, even in the way you sit and ponder a problem. It's called body language. It's an air that you create around yourself.

High Expectations

When and if those <u>expectations</u> go unmet, you quite naturally will react in ways to correct those miscalculations. And the life you actively carve out for yourself will reflect and be largely determined by those high expectations.

Low Expectations…

On the other hand, *if you see yourself as weak, physically incapable, mentally lacking, etc., guess how you're going to <u>expect</u> the world and the people in it to treat you?* And if those <u>expectations</u> go unmet, you quite naturally will react in ways to correct those miscalculations.

And the life you carve out for yourself will reflect and be largely determined by those low expectations.

So What Do You Expect?

But let's presume that, like most people I've worked with over the years, you're somewhere in between supremely self confident and infinitely lacking in confidence. If that's the case, you'll find it very helpful to spend *five minutes a day*, eyes closed, relaxed, sitting and visualizing yourself as having already reached your goals. That is to say, in your mind you should immediately travel to the "I am who I want to be right now" stage!

Building Expectations...

With the body you've always dreamed of having, see (feel, taste, smell, and hear) yourself confidently walking down the street, meeting and talking with others, effectively being the person you intend to become, RIGHT NOW! See yourself as assured, capable - fully appreciated by yourself and others. And in that 5 minutes a day you'll find that your self expectations, and so your relationship with and reactions to the world, will change, be transformed in wonderful ways. And as your expectations grow and improve, your relationships, reactions, and your quality of life will improve as well.

Expect A Miracle?

I used to chuckle at Televangelist Oral Roberts when he always ended his broadcast by telling his flock to "expect a miracle." Now that I've learned the value of expectations, I find myself in complete agreement with Roberts (along with Maxwell Maltz, Norman Vincent Peale, etc). I now realize that when you upgrade your expectations, you naturally, automatically upgrade the quality of your life…simultaneously!

Arrogant Enough…

In the words of the great Australian (former world record holding) miler Herb Elliott "*you must be arrogant enough to think you can (break the world record in this case), and humble enough to actually do it.*" If you don't expect to reach your goals you'll never be able to hang in there and persist long enough to do it. On the other hand, you must humble yourself enough to pay the price.

With this unique combination, you'll inch closer and closer to your goals every day, every week, every month, until, when it is all said and done, you're living the life you've always dreamed of living, and serving as a role model for others who would love to follow in your footsteps, but don't yet know how to connect all the dots, how to become a winner…every day, for the rest of your life.

The Formula...

So the formula goes like this. Your self image generates your expectations. Your expectations in turn create honest and natural actions and reactions to the world around you. And the way you interact with the world, will define your life. So do it right! Do it NOW! But no matter what you do...DO IT!

So Mom And Dad, When It Comes To Childhood Obesity You Have Several Options To Choose From…!

So you're a parent with two young kids, twins in fact named Jason and Jennifer, age four and five respectively. Both are happy and healthy kids that you've raised with careful tender love, care, and affection. But you've been reading about what they're now calling the epidemic in childhood obesity, and how the problem has increased over 300% in the last two decades, and obesity in general is threatening to bypass tobacco as the number one preventable cause of death in the US today.

You fear now that Jason's and Jennifer's affinity for fast food and computerized video games is going to result in the kids becoming obese and suffering from all the problems that go hand in hand with kids being overweight/obese. You absolutely don't want them to be subjected to that kind of treatment from peers, who we all know can be extremely mean even at a very young age.

Being a pro-active parent you begin to search the available literature on how to prevent childhood obesity before it begins. You go to the library, the book store, the internet and what do you find? Here's a potpourri of the prescriptions that are currently out there on the market for you to choose from.

- You can depend on your doctor and the AMA (American Medical Association) to become inspired with the idea that losing weight is primarily a function of changing lifestyles and habits that lead to the problem in the first place. Basically they tell you that you have to reduce your kid's calorie intake, and increase their physical activity level, and that habits and lifestyles are the culprits or the heroes when it comes to weight control in kids or adults. So make sure they get thirty to sixty minutes of active play every day, and cut the junk foods out of their diet... even though the television ads show and tell them how much fun (you deserve a break today) and delicious they are. The problem is they tell you to do it without telling how to motivate your kids to actually do it.

- You can depend on the Health Club to inspire your kids to increase their protein intake, decrease their carbohydrates, and design a circuit training (a combination of weights and aerobics) routine like their adult club members employ on a weekly basis.

And the membership will run you about $49 per month, or $600 per year. But if it works, it's worth it, right? But I suggest checking out their success rates before signing your kids up.

- You can depend on the Park District and sign your kids up to participate in a sport each summer, fall, winter, and spring. The hope is that your kids will get hooked on athletics, and in the process they burn all the excess calories running up and down the soccer field or the basketball court. They also have less time to vegetate on the TV or the computer if they're participating in sports. But what if they prefer the cello?

- You can depend on the school that Jason and Jennifer both attend to eliminate the junk food in the vending machines and to teach a good Physical Education classes. After all it has a very good reputation in the neighborhood, so you could just place the fate of your kids in the hands of the school system and hope that they'll learn all about being physically active and eating right. Yes you could do that…right?

- In short you could depend on the system and lots of other people and programs to help your kids avoid the modern, high tech obesity trap. Or you could take the bull by the horns yourself and teach your own kids to perform pull ups because you know that people who can pull their own weight are never obese, and people who are obese can never do pull ups. So, the ability to perform pull ups and the possibility of being obese are mutually exclusive, and are never found in the same person. You know this from observing kids in gym class back when you were in school. It was always the relatively lean kids who could perform pull ups, and always the heavy kids who weighed to much to pull their own weight, and were inevitably embarrassed by any reference to the old pull up bar. So the choice is up to you. Do you depend on someone else, or do it yourself (pull your own weight) in about five minutes a week?

The Gym Teacher And His Four Big Challenges

As a former Physical Education teacher who taught and coached in public schools for seventeen years before moving over in the writing profession, I've found the frenzy and frustration over the so-called childhood obesity epidemic in the US to be very interesting. The time and money being spent by panels of experts researching, documenting, prescribing, and promoting one simple solution – eat less and exercise more – is astonishing. And the only thing that's more astonishing is the lack of success that the experts and the promoters are experiencing in the wake. The kids seem to be oblivious to the message, while buying into fast foods and video games promos instead.

My True Confession

Now, before I make the following observations I have to confess I am personally no expert. I'm no exercise physiologist or nutritionist, and I have no PhD behind my name. In fact if you checked it out you'd find that I was pretty much of a C student for the largest part of my academic career. So what I'm about to say is nothing more, and nothing less than an observation I made back in my teaching and coaching days that looks like an utterly simple and natural solution to me. See if you agree.

I noticed in my gym classes that kids who could perform pull ups were noticeably leaner and relatively stronger than the kids who were unable to perform pull ups. You may have noticed the same thing back when you were back in school.

Anyway, as you can imagine, over seventeen years, I taught thousands of kids, and using my own experience as the basis, I would say that you can go to the bank on my simple pull up observation. In fact I recently turned the observation into what I call my Wall A, Wall B Story. Check it out.

Wall A, Wall B Story

Go into any school gym in the country and ask all the students who can perform at least one pull up to stand by wall A, and all those who can't to stand by wall B. What you'll then see is what I call The Great Fitness Divide, with all the relatively lean and strong students on wall A, and all the relatively overweight and weak students on wall B.

My conclusion? Start very young (grades K, 1, or 2) before most kids have a chance to gain too much excess weight, and teach them to be able to perform pull ups. Then make them understand that if they maintain their

106

ability to perform pull ups, they'll always be relatively lean and strong, and they'll never be much overweight and/or weak, or subjected to all the related embarrassments and problems.

In other words, if you can do pull-ups, you can't be obese, and the more pull-ups you can do, the leaner you have to be naturally, as a matter of course. There's no choice. Isn't it about time to teach all our kids from sea to shining sea to Pull Their Own Weight?

The Four Challenges

I also recognize that what I'm saying here doesn't sound like statistics laden, scientific research. And it's not. It's simply something that I observed with my own two Physical Educator's eyeballs during my seventeen years in the teaching profession. However, I'm sure enough of this observation that I will now make the following four challenges to the experts out across the US.

- I challenge **physical educators** around the country to stand up and disagree with my simple pull ups observation. In other words, I don't think you will be able to find a gym teacher who hasn't seen the same thing that I've seen and described here. It's absolutely common knowledge in this profession that kids who are overweight can't perform pull ups, and kids who can perform pull ups are not overweight. They are and always will be mutually exclusive.

- However knowing how much the experts love numbers, I also challenge **exercise physiologists** around the country to perform one simple experiment. Go into a local high school, a junior high school, and an elementary school and test the student's body composition using the simple caliper method. Then have the gym teacher divide his kids into Wall A and Wall B. Finally compare the body compositions of the Wall A students to the Wall B students. I predict that you'll see a very significant difference between the two, and that <u>none of the wall A kids will be obese</u>. The experts will like that.

- To take this line of reasoning one step further using the same data, compare the body compositions of the kids who can perform one pull up to those who can perform five, ten, fifteen, and twenty pull ups. What you will find, to no gym teacher's surprise, is that more pull ups a student can do, the lower their body fat will be. With these two experiments **overseen by experts**, everyone will have all the statistics and the data they need to substantiate numerically what every gym teacher in the country already knows, which is that the ability to perform pull ups and obesity are never found in the same person.

- Finally I challenge **the media**, both print and electronic to publicize the following letter (in the appendix at the end of the book) that has been totally and completely ignored by the Chicago Tribune. For people across the country to understand this simple solution, the media must decide to tell them about it, or it'll remain a gym teacher's secret forever.

- With this information in hand, the next logical step is to recognize that all we have to do to eliminate childhood obesity in this country is to teach our kids, starting at the kindergarten level, to be able to perform pull ups. Once they've cultivated that ability, they are armed with their very own functional antidote to obesity for the rest of their lives, so long as they maintain that new found ability.

Action or Procrastination...The Choice Is Yours

Now the next question is aimed at the reader. Do you want to wait for the experts to generate the numbers before you take action on this idea? If so, that's your prerogative. Sooner or later you may see those researched statistics and at that point you can roll right into action.

On the other hand maybe you're one of those people who say, "You know this makes too much sense, I know exactly what this guy is talking about. I just can't believe that nobody has pointed it out before. I don't need permission from some group of experts to act on common sense. Let's start teaching pull ups today. What's the cheapest and most cost effective way to get started?" If you're a member of the latter group, read on because what I'm about to talk about is for you...the action oriented person who thinks for himself or herself.

But I'm getting ahead of myself here. Allow me to give you a little background so that you can fully understand and appreciate the utter simplicity and naturalness of this user friendly solution to the childhood obesity problem in this country. Let's talk for a moment about Mother Nature and how she set things up in the first place.

"The Simple 12 Step Program That Stops Childhood Obesity In Its Tracks, Naturally!"

Although I completely agree with anyone who claims that any one of the previously discussed exercises will serve as a solid functional antidote against childhood obesity, I also believe that none of them is as user friendly as the simple pull up. Allow me to explain why I feel this way.

It's Cheap

First and foremost the equipment, a pull up bar is cheap, it takes up almost no room in the house, the gym, the garage, or wherever you choose to place it. That means almost anyone can afford the equipment, and they could find a place to locate it if they wanted to do so.

Everyone Knows What It Is

Second, everyone knows what a pull up is. This is not true of the other exercises. I mean walk into the closest mall and ask ten people what a pull up is and they'll all know. On the other hand ask ten people to explain dips, hand stand push ups, or any of the others and there's no telling what you'll hear.

Logistics Are Easy and There's No Exposure To Injury

Third, I do agree that all the others can be taught and learned, but the logistics of teaching pull ups are easier than any of them. For example, rope climbing done wrong can easily produce rope burns and injury. Super Man Push Ups done incorrectly can jeopardize a participant's lower back. Hand stand push ups require a great sense of balance along with strength and lightness. Sissy squat stands are really hard to find and can be relatively expensive. And dips require a dip station or a set of parallel bars, and some adaptive equipment that will allow an unable participant to learn to do them.

On the other hand, using the height adjustable bar, and the leg assisted technique, pull ups are easily taught and learned without exposing participants to potential injury or requiring logistically challenging and expensive adaptive techniques. In simple terms, teaching kids to perform pull ups is easy, inexpensive, and takes very little time. Yes you heard that right. *In about five minutes of work each week* almost any child can be taught to do pull ups.

I've Seen Lots Of Kids Succeed

Perhaps most importantly, I can say all this with confidence because I've had four years of personal experience teaching elementary school age (K-3) kids to move from Wall B (those who are unable to perform pull ups) to Wall A (those who are able to perform pull ups) in a program that we called PULL YOUR OWN WEIGHT. From this experience I can attest that if you start 'em young, almost all kids can be taught to perform pull ups. At the risk of being repetitious, with my own two eyes I've witnessed lots of kids learning to perform pull ups using a very simple and inexpensive technique that anyone (no you don't have to be a Physical Educator) can use to get the job done.

A Winning, Highly Promoteable Phrase

The final plug I would like to make here in favor of pull ups over all the rest is that the phrase PULL YOUR OWN WEIGHT has a very positive ring to it, and connotes a variety of good things that make it almost as American as red, white, and blue, motherhood, baseball, and apple pie, all rolled into one. It offers anyone who's interested in doing so, a very simple way to promote regular exercise habits, good eating habits, avoidance of tobacco alcohol, drugs, while chipping away in a very visible and concrete way at the problem of childhood obesity, adolescent obesity, and eventually adult obesity in our modern high tech, fast food, couch potato based society.

Anyone Can Teach/Learn It

The simple fact of the matter is that those who can physically pull their own weight (perform pull ups) cannot be obese. And those who are obese, cannot pull their own weight. The two are mutually exclusive and you don't find one in the same package as the other. So let's teach everyone to perform pull ups safely, predictably, inexpensively, and naturally. With all that said, I'll now tell you about the simple 12 step program through which anyone can learn to pull their own weight in a predictable period of time. Check it out.

Here's The 12 Step PYOW Program In A Nutshell

1. **Read the Johnny and Jamal story** (see the appendix) to your child in order to set the stage and give 'em a context in which to understand the Pull Your Own Weight program.

2. **Introduce the Height Adjustable Pull Up Bar/Leg Assisted, Jump Pull Up Technique** by demonstrating it, and allowing the kids to try it. They'll all quickly discover that the strategy is to show all participants how to succeed right from the get go, and to give them a way to progress regularly, and feel good about what they are accomplishing...in public.

3. **Determine/Record The Participant's Correct Starting Point** by adjusting the bar level to a point where they can perform at least eight pull ups, but not more than twelve. The idea here is to do eight repetitions in the first work out, nine in the second, ten in the third, eleven in the fourth, and twelve in the fifth. When the participant performs twelve pull

ups at this height, the bar is moved up one inch and the entire eight to twelve routine is performed all over again.

4. **Determine/Record the level** at which the child will eventually run out of leg assistance, the point at which he or she is doing regular pull-ups, and designate that level as the participant's END GOAL. Then **Count the number of links** from their starting point to their end goal, and multiply that number by five in order to determine approximately *how many workouts it will take* to achieve the end goal. Depending on how many workouts per week you do (maximum of three) you should also determine *how many weeks it will take* to reach the end goal, mark that date of their projected final work out on the calendar and aim to finish up by that date.

5. **Do workout number one** with the child performing eight pull-ups at their designated starting point. When they're done, make sure and give the child a high five, a smile, and a pat on the back so they know, and all their peers know that you're proud of them.

6. On the PYOW chart, **record each workout date, the level** at which the workout was done, along with the number of pull-ups (between eight and twelve) the child did on that day. Then set a date for workout number two.

7. If you have multiple children participating, **make sure that they are all rooting for each other**, giving each other high fives, and patting each other on the back. This strategy effectively promotes self competition, winning almost performances every time, children experiencing joy in other's success, and teamwork.

8. If possible, find five or ten minutes to **talk with the kids** about their feelings and the various lessons that can be learned from this project (i.e. getting stronger through regular workouts over a period of time, eating right, getting sufficient rest, the fact that nobody else can do the work for them, you have to do it for yourself, how avoiding tobacco, alcohol, and drugs makes you strong, not weak, and lots more that's discussed in detail in a later chapter.)

9. **Follow the inch by inch strategy all the way to the END GOAL.** When the child has accomplished the goal they should receive a material reward of some sort (a "Wall A" T-Shirt or baseball hat, etc). From this point forward they are allowed to do as many pull-ups in each workout as they can do. We called this achievement...PASSING YOUR BAR EXAM.

10. From this point forward, **one workout a week will probably allow them to maintain their ability** to perform pull-ups, and to remain on Wall-A. But if their performance begins to slip, say from twelve pull-ups one week down to ten the next week, that's a WARNING SIGN that they need to adjust something. It could be their diet if they're picking up weight, or it could be the amount of rest they're getting at night. It could be they'll have to increase their workouts per week back up to two or even three in some cases. But quick and easy adjustments will allow them to maintain the level of performance they've cultivated and to stay firmly on Wall-A for as long as they choose to do so.

11. Now if a child can perform a certain number of regular pull-ups **but still wants to be leaner**, all they have to do is to increase the number of pull-ups they can do and the leanness will follow as a matter of course, naturally. In other words, more pull-ups means more strength (muscle mass), or less body weight, or a combination of both…any one of which indicates an improvement in body composition, the fact that the child is becoming leaner.

12. **Understand that the Golden Rule of PYOW** (those who can do pull-ups can't be obese, or those who are obese, can't do pull-ups) is just as true for teenagers and adults as it is for elementary school kids. So, Mom and Dad, or big brother or sister, if you want to be a model for your elementary age participant then have at it. There's nothing better for your child than to see you walking the walk right along with them.

Recognize That You're Building More Than Strength

Understand at the initial stages you're building much more than upper body strength. *You're also building in the expectation of success.* So it's critical at the initial stages that regular progress is achieved, and recognized with high fives, etc. The child should feel good about doing his pull ups, and *even look forward to the opportunity to do them*, because (s)he is not allowed to do more than three workouts a week. Actually progress will occur with only two workouts a week if you want to restrict it that much. But again the restriction makes it special, and not something they can do any old time.

So in the big picture, as you raise the bar, and increase the workload, along with the child's sense of "I can do this," the bar will eventually become high enough that they run out of leg assistance and they'll achieve the goal of pulling their own weight in a conventional sense. But again, there's still more going on here than meets the eye.

Self Confidence And Motivation Is Built Into This Program

Now that sense of "I can do this," the sense that "I can try something a little bit harder than I did last time and still expect to succeed," is called confidence, self esteem, self worth, etc., and it's crucial to anyone's growth potential in any endeavor whether it's pull ups, a high school degree, or succeeding in business. *If you're scared to try, you're doomed to fail.*

The possibility of success is often stopped in its tracks by a person's own inability to take a chance, by a person's own fear of failure. The fact of the matter is, anyone who is psychologically intimidated by failure has effectively doomed himself, stunted his own growth, and guaranteed his own failure. In order to grow and to succeed in anything you have to have confidence enough to try something a little new, something a little bit harder than last time...and you must "expect to be able to do this." Failing to try, guarantees failure!

What Happens When Progress Stalls?

And if you reach a plateau where progress has stalled, you must be able to step back and figure out a way to start it moving again. Using pull ups as an example, you may have to adjust the amount of rest you're getting in between workouts, add some calorie burning aerobics to your routine, or modify the quantity or quality of the food you're eating to drop a little weight, and just watch as progress kicks back into gear as the result of your adjustment.

Now let me ask, how valuable is it to learn these kinds of lessons in a hands on kind of way, at an early age? If you say "it's real important," you see what I mean when I say the lessons you'll learn from a pull-up bar go well beyond eliminating obesity.

A Natural Antidote To Peer Pressure

This self confidence thing by the way is that inner sense of strength and self worth that allows a child to think for himself and to avoid caving into peer pressure in situations where that needs to occur. A child who lacks that genuine sense of self confidence, is the child who is swayed by the group into doing things that he knows down deep, he should be avoiding. But psychologically they can't afford to buck the crowd and to be called un-cool, etc. Inner strength weathers the peer pressure storm, and allows a child to stick with doing things that make him strong, and to actively avoid things that make him weak.

Why Concentrate On Pull Ups Alone?

I've one had a personal trainer friend named Linda say, "Why in the world do you concentrate on pull ups alone when it's common knowledge that a variety of exercises is necessary to any well conceived fitness plan? I mean to start with, you have to have aerobic work, anaerobic work, and flexibility too, right? And pull ups are only one small piece of the anaerobic part of the puzzle. Your program is so linear, so singular, so hopelessly incomplete that it borders on being silly."

Ever Hear of Sir Roger Bannister?

My first response was to inform Linda that nobody ever said OPYOW was a comprehensive fitness plan. In fact it's the polar opposite. Then I asked Linda her opinion of Sir Roger Bannister, the first human to crack the four-minute barrier in the mile run. He was concentrated like a laser, on tenths of seconds, in one event…the mile run. What about the legendary Muhammed Ali who concentrated only on boxing, and now Tiger Woods who concentrates on golf alone. "What's the difference," I asked Linda.

They Have Sophisticated Regiments

"The difference of course," she said "is that all those athletes have sophisticated fitness regiments. They did all kinds of things to improve in the mile, the boxing ring, and the golf swing. I've heard that Tiger Woods can bench press over 250 lbs! Now that's pretty impressive for a golfer," she said. They're concentrated on their sport, but their diversified in their workouts. Whatever it takes to better themselves, they do it."

Thanks Linda...

I thanked Linda for that fine explanation, and then I told her that we treat pull ups in the same way that Bannister treated the mile, Ali treated boxing, and Woods treats golf. "It's the acid test, the bottom line, and the prime motivator that guides, informs, and justifies regular work, good eating and resting habits, and avoiding tobacco, alcohol, and drugs so you'll stronger, not weaker on the pull up bar," I said. "And if progress slows, then you'd better adjust one or more of these factors in order to jump start your progress," I said. "It's about as simple as that."

A Customized Experiment

In other words, to a certain degree, getting stronger on the pull up bar (OPYOW) becomes a customized, hands on experiment designed to help each participant discover what it takes to improve week after week, month after month, year after year? In this sense, like Bannister's mile, Ali's boxing, and Woods' golf, OPYOW is non restrictive and it encourages all participants to do whatever it takes, short of performance enhancing drugs, to develop and maintain the ability to do pull ups. If you do you'll remain lean and strong for the rest of your life.

Instead, The Short Term Goal...

Instead it says the short-term goal for OPYOW participants is to improve regularly, workout after workout, week after week, month after month, and hopefully year after year. On the other hand, the long-term goal is to develop and maintain the ability to do real live pull ups. And in order to be naturally immunized against obesity for the rest of your life, just always maintain the ability to do pull ups.

A Different Twist at the Same Question

Then I had a different friend pose a similar question in a little different way. Sandy W from Fayetteville, AK said, "Why does it have to be pull ups? I hate pull ups and so does everyone else that I know. Why can't the acid test be a twenty five inch vertical jump, hand stand push ups, dips, or any one of a number of things I could mention off the top of my head? Why do you insist on pull ups? Why?

Let me answer by saying I'm not aiming to upset anyone's apple cart with OPYOW, especially Sandy W's. And of course she's right is contending that a good vertical jump, hand stand push ups, or dips pay you to be both strong and light, just like pull ups. And there are certainly other possibilities that you could point out ranging from a superman push up to a seven minute mile that would serve the same purpose.

They All Share One Thing in Common

Notice however that all theses acid tests share one factor in common. They all use the participant's own body weight as the primary resistance factor instead of weights, plates, rubber bands, and computers. In other words if you choose from any activity in which the participant's own body weight is the primary resistance factor and you will continue minimizing your body fat as your performance improves. Under such conditions they (performance and body fat) are inversely related, and thus reflective of one another.

Why Focus on One Flavor When There Are Many...

So what Sandy wants to know is why we've decided to concentrate on one flavor of exercise (pull ups) when ere are really many flavors to choose from? And to be honest, when the decision was made, there were several things taken into consideration, beginning with the fact that pull ups are simple. Everyone understands them and associates them with strength.

Second, you don't have to be an Exercise Physiologist to understand that kids who can do pull ups ARE NEVER OBESE. You can make that observation on the playground, or in any gym class with your own two eyes. It's no secret. And finally we chose pull ups because they fit the phrase Pull Your Own Weight like a glove.

Thanks Sandy

But thanks to Sandy, we've now addressed the fact that there are numerous different flavors of OPYOW to choose from if you also hate pull ups. Constructive criticism is and always will be welcome in this camp.

About Nutrition, Aerobics, Rest, Avoiding Tobacco, Alcohol, Drugs & Flexibility

In this section I'm going to stray a little bit from our PYOW path in order to talk about several issues that generally fall under the category of physical fitness. That's not to say that the subject matter so far has not been fitness related, because it certainly has. But the intention of this book has not been to present a comprehensive fitness program, and it does not pretend to do so. This book is nothing more and nothing less than a simple, naturalistic, functional solution to childhood obesity. But since comprehensive fitness subjects are related, there are several things I want to mention now

The topics I want to talk about here, in a very general sense, are nutrition, aerobics, rest, avoiding tobacco, alcohol, and drugs, and flexibility. And I'm going to talk about them only in so far as they are helpful when it comes to children learning to improve themselves on the pull up bar.

Ok, first things first. It's much easier to develop strength if you eat right. It's also much easier to drop fat weight when you eat right. And make no mistake about it, a pull up bar knows when you gain or lose muscle or fat and it pays you or it punishes the performer immediately with performance improvements or failures. You see like life in general, a pull up bar pays you to be strong and light.

That is not to say that you won't make good progress without watching your diet. In fact I'd be willing to bet that you will. But what happens if you hit a plateau and progress starts getting harder and harder to produce? When this happens, and it almost always does, you have to be able to take a step back and assess the situation, make the necessary adjustments, and continue on with your progress. Now when making that kind of assessment there are several factors you will want to take into consideration including nutrition, aerobics, rest, avoiding tobacco, alcohol, and drugs, and flexibility.

For example, you could stand back and ask yourself "Am I getting enough protein to build my muscles up naturally. If the answer is no, the solution to the may be that you need to add some meat, fish, or poultry to your diet in order to increase the protein necessary to build your strength and muscles. You could also add vegetable protein in the form of soy or certain kinds of beans/legumes.

On the other hand you may think that in order to improve on the pull up bar, you must lose as much excess body weight (fat) as possible, and in order to do that you'll have to cut some calories, but don't cut from the protein side of the ledger. You could achieve this desirable end by simply drinking more water, increasing your fruit and vegetable intake, or you could replace the candy bar and sweetened drink snacks with an apple or a banana. And whatever you do avoid the golden arches, their friends and fellow members of the fast/junk food industry because you'll gain calories by just walking in the door and reading the menu. The long and the short of it is eat right, drop some unnecessary pounds, reduce the workload (your body weight) and your progress will jump right back on the first train going north.

Now since we're not intending or claiming to be a nutrition book here, I want to keep things basic and to avoid confusing a simple issue by giving you what I like to call my *Top Ten Strong Foods* (foods that help you get strong and independent), and my *Top Ten Weak Foods* (yes, that's food that will make you weak and dependent) that can serve as a quick and easy reference, and help you to develop the ability to perform more and more pull ups, getting stronger and lighter by the day, by the week, and by the month. Here they are.

The Top Ten Strong Foods

1. Meat (chicken and fish are both better than red meat)
2. Raw Vegetables
3. Raw Fruit
4. Eggs
5. Milk (Skim)
6. Whole Grain Cereal
7. Soy Products
8. Cheese (Low Fat)
9. Nuts
10. Water (it's hard to drink enough of H_2O)

The Top Ten Weak Foods

1. Pizza
2. Soda Pop
3. French Fries
4. Candy Bars
5. Ice Cream
6. Cookies
7. Cake
8. Fried Anything
9. High Fat Meat
10. White Bread

One final note, if you insist on addressing nutrition in terms of *a diet*, check out the incredibly easy, *Australian Outback Diet* in the next chapter, and follow it.

Add Aerobics To Your Weekly Schedule

When you stand back and make your assessment, there are several other adjustments that will want to take into account, one of them being the possibility of adding some aerobic activity to your weekly schedule. Now since aerobics are basically endurance activities like walking, running, swimming, and biking, you may be tempted to ask what they have to do with pull up performance? Since they are generally associated with cardio or heart strength, how does adding aerobics improve your pull up performance?

The answer is that because of their endurance characteristics, aerobic activities burn more calories per unit time than anything else you can do. And burning calories will help reduce fat weight and improve pull up performance quickly. For example, you will burn lots more calories in a leisurely ten minute walk around the block than in a ten to twenty second bout on the pull up bar because you are walking for lots more time. Sure the pull ups are much harder, more intense, and more difficult, but exhaustion occurs so quickly in high intensity exercise that you don't have a chance to burn many calories.

Now it's basically true that increasing your strength, increases your muscle mass, which increases your metabolism and burns more calories. But in terms of calories burned in a given exercise session, it's impossible to beat aerobics. So the moral of the story here is that if your pull up progress stalls, adding aerobics to your weekly schedule, burning more calories, and dropping some weight, is one adjustment that could help you get back on track.

Getting Sufficient Rest

A third factor that will affect your pull up performance is rest, and I mean this in two different ways. First you should limit your workouts to no more than three per week, and two will often produce similar results. Either way you should avoid working out on consecutive days because you need at least forty eight hours of rest in order to recover from your workout and allow your muscles to build the desired new strength. Working out on consecutive days you'll discover are actually counterproductive.

The other rest issue you should be aware of is the amount of sleep you get at night. Research has proven that a child needs at least eight hours of sleep per night in order to grow and to perform up to par. In other words, if you're staying up late for any reason - to do your homework or to watch Television – you could be holding yourself back on the pull up bar. So when it comes to rest, get enough of it between workouts, and get enough sleep at night and you'll help yourself to get stronger and stronger on the pull up bar.

So when you're standing back and making your assessment, don't forget to take rest into consideration. Getting enough of it can make lots of difference in your performance in lots of things, including the pull up bar.

Tobacco, Alcohol, and Drugs

The next topic I want to address in this section is the use of tobacco, alcohol, and drugs. Yes, I know that these are common in many homes and many neighborhoods across the country, and that many kids are exposed to them on a regular basis. However the one point that I want to make here is simply that THE USE OF TOBACCO, ALCOHOL, AND DRUGS MAKES YOU WEAK AND DEPENDENT NOT STRONG AND INDEPENDENT! If you really want to be weak, the fastest way to get there is to abuse your body by using tobacco, alcohol, and drugs. Let me add that I've known lots of kids who want to "be bad." But I've never ever met a kid who wants to be weak. Have you?

Some may say "What about steroids? Those are drugs and they make you strong don't they?" And I will tell you that the strength that they produce is only temporary. But in the long run, steroids render the user weak and dependent just like cigarettes, booze, heroin and crack cocaine. So if your aim is to get strong and to be able to do lots of pull ups for years to come, steer clear of tobacco, alcohol, and drugs, because they make you weak and dependent, not strong and independent...period!

Flexibility and Stretching

The fifth and final topic I want to talk about here is one that is related to a comprehensive fitness program, but really has little effect on your ability to perform pull ups. That subject is flexibility which is gained from stretching. Am I an advocate of stretching? Yes I am. Do I practice what I preach on this issue? I must confess that I have always had a hard time walking the walk when it comes to stretching and flexibility.

I do however know the benefits of having muscles with a sufficient amount of elasticity, including the relaxation factor, the injury prevention factor, and the anti-aging factor promoted by a good stretching habit, by having flexible muscles – particularly in the hamstrings which play a strong in preventing lower back pain.

So what do I actually do? I stretch when I find time, and it's usually a stretching of my hamstrings, and my back muscles that feels good, kind of like your pet dog or pet cat who stretch their limbs after waking from an afternoon nap. That's what I do, and at 57 years of existence, I'm probably not going to change much on this issue.

Anyway, if you want to cultivate a comprehensive program in your life, include some stretching in your week. On the other hand if you just want to avoid becoming overweight for the rest of your life, it's much more important to develop the ability to perform pull ups and to maintain that ability. Do that and you'll never ever be obese...period!

The Incredibly Easy, Australian Outback Diet That Totally Ignores Calories, Carbs, Fat Grams, and Bathroom Scales Too

So, when you want to drop excess weight, what do you count? Calories? Carbs? Fat grams? Weight Watcher's Points? Or do you do like the Australians in the Outback who wrap 'em all in one big package and count *consecutive g'days, g'weeks, g'months, g'years, g'lifetimes?*

You see to have g'days and g'weeks automatically results in…

- reduced calories,
- reduced body fat,
- improved body composition,
- improved functional capacity,
- increased energy,
- increased confidence,
- and increased performance in almost everything you do
- without ever getting lost in the numerical detail of calorie, carb, or fat gram counting that makes dieting a frustrating waste of time for most humans,

- without depending on a scale to tell you if you're winning or losing the war.
- Not only that but, b'days result in precisely the opposite

By concentrating on t'day (yesterday is dead and gone, and t'morrow has yet to arrive), stringing consecutive g'days together into g'weeks and g'months, you're creating g'habits that in turn create g'lifestyles that win...naturally. It's a common sense way to look at weight control that contradicts the modern tendency to get lost in the numerical detail, missing the forest for the trees. Australian outback *g'day counters* are operating in the big picture, and they know that weight control is not all that hard if you can just string weeks and months worth of g'days together into a g'lifestyle that works for you.

Now what does a g'day look like you ask? Here's a (baker's) dozen specific characteristics that characterize a g'day. You may even want to add a few things to this list. But, if you do these things, you've just had one g'day. Now check 'em out, see what you think.

- First and foremost, forget the short term diet mentality. If you don't plan on making this a lifetime habit, then it's not even worth fiddling with.

- Concentrate on t'day because yesterday's gone, and t'morrow has yet to arrive. If you take care of t'day you won't look back and regret yesterday, while t'morrow will look infinitely better from where you now stand t'day.
- Eat three good meals each day, and breakfast is the most important one
- Never feel stuffed (in other words always eat reasonable portions)
- If you snack in between meals, snack on healthy foods
- Drink plenty of water (minimally eight 8oz glasses) each day
- Get some exercise
- Get sufficient rest at night
- Avoid tobacco, alcohol, and drugs
- Stop weighing yourself...if you must, never do it more than once a week
- Stop counting calories, carbs, fat grams, or weight watcher points
- Instead, count g'days, and string 'em into g'weeks, g'months, and g'years
- Keep a daily G'day Journal for at least 100 consecutive g'days

- Always remember that your main goal is to cultivate g'habits that will naturally (without having to work at it) underwrite a g'lifestyle and finally make weight control easy and natural for you.

Three Specific Instances

Fifty Out of Fifty Chose Pull-Ups

    A second grade teacher (Dari Spotten) had invited a rural second grade teacher to bring her class to our school (Jefferson Elementary) in order to get a taste of what an inner city school is like. The day was tightly planned right down to the minute, and the last two things on the agenda were recess and Pull Your Own Weight. But as the day came to a close the teachers both recognized that they only had time for one of these activities, so they put it up for a vote...recess or PYOW? I'm here to tell you that 50 out of 50 second graders chose to do pull-ups over recess. Who said kids can't learn to love pull-ups?

Paying for the Opportunity to do Pull Ups

    At Jefferson School back in the nineties we had an annual fun night, which was a PTA sponsored fundraiser where parents and teachers would donate a dish of something to eat, and booths would be set up all around the gym with various games that would attract and amuse the kids. Access to the food and the games was accomplished by purchasing tickets from the PTA table for a quarter a ticket.

On one of these occasions the PTA decided that a pull-up bar was going to be one of the booths, and that yours truly would be the official counter of pull-ups. Believe it not that fun night went on for over two hours and I had kid standing in line eight to ten deep, **PAYING for the opportunity** to get on the pull-up bar in order to show their proud parents how strong they'd become. At the end of the evening I had lost my voice from counting pull-ups. And if kids can learn to love pull-ups, why can't they learn to love reading, writing, and arithmetic too? My bet is that they can.

No Way! That'll Make Me Weak...

I was talking to a kindergarten class about Pull Your Own Weight when one little boy in the back raised his hand and proceeded to tell me and the rest of the class "Coach, my uncle Willie tried to talk me into smoking a cigarette last night, but I said NO WAY! That will make me WEAK!" That may have been the single most gratifying moment of my entire seventeen-year teaching career. It goes to show this program goes well beyond preventing childhood obesity, and proving that **EVEN KINDERGARTNERS GET IT.**

An Open Letter to Physical Educators: A Golden Opportunity Is Knockin'

In educational circles these days, subjects like reading, math, and science generally get top billing in local school districts. And at the bottom comes music, art, and physical education... often in that order. In other words, when the local budget slashers look at where they can cut educational funds and services, physical education suddenly gets an unwanted spotlight.

The Big Challenge

But interestingly enough with the recent challenge of childhood obesity getting so much media attention, physical educators suddenly have a golden opportunity to turn the tables, and transform themselves from budget cutting victims into indispensable community heroes.

That is to say, *if you can cost effectively show the kids in your classes how to naturally immunize themselves against obesity for a lifetime, without resorting to shots, pills, or special diets, (and get the local media to talk about it)* your colleagues including fellow teachers, the building principal, district administrators, the superintendent of

143

schools, the school board, and the parents will erect a statue in your image, and offer you a well earned raise in place of a pink slip.

Most Don't Know About OPYOW

The problem is, most physical educators don't know how to teach their students to naturally immunize themselves against obesity for a lifetime, without resorting to shots, pills, or special diets. In other words, most physical educators don't know about an incredibly simple, cost effective program called Operation Pull Your Own Weight that I'm about to describe in the following paragraphs.

Wall A, Wall B

However most of them will relate to the following scenario. Walk into any physical education class in the USA and ask all the kids who are able to do at least one legitimate pull up to stand by wall A. Then ask all the kids who are unable to do one pull to stand on wall B. What you'll witness is what I call the great fitness divide, with the relatively strong and trim kids standing by wall A, and the relatively weak and heavy kids standing by wall B.

The Basic Strategy

The basic strategy for Operation Pull Your Own Weight then is to systematically transport as many kids as possible from wall B to wall A, and encourage them to always maintain their newfound ability. Why? *Because people who can do pull ups can't carry much excess weight. And people who carry much excess weight, can't do pull ups.* This little observation is called the Golden Rule of Operation Pull Your Own Weight.

The Question Becomes

Presuming most physical educators can identify with this scenario, the question suddenly becomes, "How do you teach kids to pull ups when pull ups are most likely the most universally hated exercise on planet earth." The answer is, you have to recognize that it's not really pull ups that kids really hate. It's FAILING IN FRONT OF THEIR PEERS that kids really hate.

Kids who can do pull ups and who succeed in front of their peers, don't hate pull ups. *In fact they enjoy being able to tackle a difficult task like pull ups, and succeed in front of their peers.* It becomes a badge of honor, a status symbol. I personally witnessed an entire school full of kids learning to love pull ups back in the early nineties.

Here's How It Works

So how do you make pull ups accessible to all kids, and transform hated failure into joyful success? You use a simple device called a HEIGHT ADJUSTABLE PULL UP BAR (it raises and lowers in one inch increments) in conjunction with LEG ASSISTED PULL UPS (encouraging kids to jump and pull simultaneously) that allows *almost all kids to succeed on the pull up bar immediately in front of their peers*, for eight, ten, or even twelve (or more) consecutive weeks.

You simply allow kids to keep their feet on the ground, lower the bar to a point where *they can jump and pull simultaneously*, and easily perform eight leg assisted pull ups in workout # 1. In workout # 2 they're allowed to do nine pull ups. In workout # 3 ten, in # 4 eleven, and finally in workout # 5 they're allowed to do twelve pull ups.

When they're able to do 12 pull ups, *the bar is raised ONE INCH* and the whole eight to twelve routine is repeated over and over again until their pull up goal (the ability to do at least one) is reached. Sometimes it takes several months for kids to eventually run out of leg assistance and to reach the point where they're doing real live pull ups…IN FRONT OF THEIR PEERS and loving every second of it.

When they succeed, they get congratulated (high fives) by the teacher and their peers. It happens automatically, and participants learn to look forward to the entire experience. At that point pull ups become highly valued instead of despised.

Opportunity Not Obligation

At Jefferson Elementary School, in Davenport, IA where this strategy was first pioneered, pull ups were always treated as an opportunity (you got to do pull ups) not an obligation (you had to do pull ups). Kids were "allowed" to work out *only twice a week, and to do only one pull up more than they did last time*.

Strong VS Weak, Not Good VS Bad

OPYOW also took full advantage of every kid's desire to be strong and to avoid being weak…at anything. Have you ever met a child who wants to be weak at anything? And the ability to do pull ups is universally associated with being strong. In other words we never talked about avoiding obesity. We always talked about getting stronger on the pull up bar. The conversation was always positive, and we avoided negativity.

Lessons Bred Into OPYOW Participants

And how does a kid grow strong on the pull up bar? There are six simple answers to this question and teachers were constantly reinforcing them throughout the PYOW experience. In a very hands-on way kids learned that, in order to gain strength on the pull up bar they had to

- work regularly,
- eat right,
- get sufficient rest at night,
- and avoid tobacco,
- alcohol, and
- drugs...THEY MAKE YOU WEAK!

This point cannot be overstated so I'll repeat it once more. These kids were exposed week after week after week to the lessons of OPYOW which included...

- Gaining strength (on the bar) is an opportunity not a right – in other words, in this school you could be denied *the opportunity to get on pull up bar* if you failed to get your work done or you misbehaved in class...a reward for good behavior.
- You gain strength through regular work
- You gain strength by eating right
- You gain strength by getting enough rest

- *You become weak* by fooling around with tobacco, alcohol, and drugs
- Kids also learned that NOBODY CAN DO IT FOR YOU
- Kids learned to <u>tackle a difficult task and to succeed in public</u> by setting concrete goals, and growing in small, but regular, predictable increments.

Self Respect, Self Confidence, and Dignity

Interestingly enough the same principles that apply to strength gain on the pull up bar also apply to strength gain in reading, writing, arithmetic, and anything else in life. And by participating in OPYOW, kids not only immunize themselves against obesity for a lifetime, but they also develop a tangible sense of self respect, self confidence, and dignity that are cultivated most effectively when the PYOW seed is planted at a young age, and allowed to develop right on into adulthood.

A Golden Opportunity Indeed

All that with a simple, low tech, inexpensive height adjustable pull up bar. As I said previously, if you can show the students in your physical education classes how to immunize themselves against obesity for a lifetime, without having to resort to pills, shots, or special diets to do the trick, and you let the local newspaper, radio and TV stations know about it, you'll also become an indispensable member of the staff and you'll forget the budget slashers once and for all…a golden opportunity indeed.

How Every Gym Teacher In The Country Can Successfully Combat Childhood Obesity, In Class, Using Almost No Resources!

Thinking back over the seventeen years I spent teaching Physical Education and coaching various sports, one thing stands out to me as I read more and more about the obesity epidemic that's stalking our nation's kids today. During those years I noticed that kids who could perform pull ups were never overweight. And kids who were overweight could never perform pull ups. Now I know you don't have to be a gym teacher in order to notice that. It's common knowledge. It's so common in fact that I think we've overlooked it as an incredibly simple solution to childhood obesity. Let me explain.

Every Gym Teacher Knows What I'm Talking About

From this simple observation that at least every other gym teacher in the nation will recognize, I drew the following conclusion. Start young (i.e. grades k, 1, and 2) before they've had a chance to gain much excess weight, and teach them to be able to perform at least one pull up. Then teach them that as long as they maintain the ability to perform at least one pull up, they can never be much overweight. Furthermore, the more pull ups they can do, the leaner and stronger they'll be, naturally.

Now Hold Your Horses…

"But hold your horses here," you say. I can hear it all now. "How am I going to teach my students to do pull ups when 90% of them completely despise the exercise, and whenever possible, they avoid the pull up bar like the plague? This not the military or a police academy where you can force the participants to do pull ups. This is a school. How can I teach kids to do something that they'd never practice? And even if they wanted to practice (which they don't), most of my students can't do pull ups, so they couldn't practice even if they wanted to."

So How Do You Teach Kids To Love Doing Pull Ups

These are of course good questions and I wouldn't be writing this article if I wasn't pretty sure that I had a good, quick, and practical answer in hand. So here goes. The solution to the problem is to use a height adjustable pull up bar which you can create inexpensively by hanging a chain (one inch links) solidly from a height of ten feet (picture it attached to a basketball backboard), so it reaches down to approximately three feet from the floor.

This will accommodate the required height adjustment for all kids.

Now using a snap hook and a center mounted pull up bar, you can attach the bar to the chain at any height you choose. You can raise and lower the bar at one inch increments, which will allow every student in your class to find a level where they can perform at least eight LEG ASSISTED PULL UPS. That is to say you can find a level where every student succeeds in front of their peers. Failure is not part of this program.

Student's Inch Their Way To Success

The strategy is to allow students to work out two to three times per week and increase their repetitions from eight to nine, ten, eleven, and twelve reps. When they can do twelve repetitions at a particular height, *you move the bar up one inch* and begin the whole eight to twelve rep routine all over again. What you'll witness is kids "inching" their way up the chain over time, until eventually they run out of leg assistance. At that point they'll have learned to do real live pull ups, a feat that most of 'em could never do before you took the time to teach them how.

Emphasizing Self Competition

It's important to emphasize self competition over competition with other students. Every student is different, and they will start at various starting points and finish at various times. But the key ingredient is that each student makes visible progress regularly. It's important they see that they are better this week than last week, better this month than last month, which means that if they persist, they will reach the goal of being able to physically pull their own weight.

Some Will Need To Make Adjustments

Now in order to reach this end goal, some kids will have to adjust their nutritional intake and lose a little weight. Others may want to add some calorie burning aerobic work to accomplish a similar goal. And still others may want to experiment with the time of day they when work out, or the amount of sleep they get at night. Regardless, encourage them to do whatever they need to do (short of anabolic steroids) to get their chin up to the bar without needing of leg assistance.

Interestingly enough, you will find that the kids will make those adjustments naturally, on their own because when it's presented right, public success is built into the program right from the get go. And as successes are piled on top of successes in very thin slices, they add up to big successes, and the feeling that *they can try something a little bit harder in front of the other kids and still expect to succeed* will become more and more prevalent and resilient with each new workout.

Self Confidence Will Win The Day

Before you know it, the self esteem and self confidence that comes from succeeding in public will be visible in the way the student approaches all kinds of new tasks, from the pull up bar to memorizing their multiplication tables. When that "yes I can" attitude is firmly in place and has permeated every pore, you the gym teacher will have done much more than giving them a functional tool with which to avoid obesity for the rest of their life...which in itself is no small feat today.

You will also have given those students an inner strength that will carry them through school, through the workplace, through the ups and downs of modern day family life. You will effectively give them the green light that will help them battle their way through the challenges that life inevitably offers, and the persistence to come out the other side with a smile on their face and a cup half full instead of half empty. And if you do, you will be the best teacher these kids will ever know. Not too bad for teaching kids to do pull ups, wouldn't you agree?

So...

What Should The Gym Teacher's Goal Be?

I suggest that you find a starting place for every member of your class at the beginning of the school year. You'll discover right off the bat that some will be able to do regular pull ups, while others will need to use the leg assisted technique to learn how. With this thought in mind, the gym teacher's goal in my view should be to monitor the percentage of kids who can do regular pull ups, and to make sure that percentage is always going up.

For example if ten percent of your class can do real live pull ups at the beginning of the year, it would be great if fifteen could do it by semester time, and twenty percent by the end of the school year...although you may do much better than that. In short, the closer we get to having all students vaccinated against obesity by maintaining the ability to physically pull their own weight, the closer we will be to winning the war on obesity.

How To Organize A Pull Your Own Weight Program In Physical Education Class

If I were still a physical education teacher today, and I wanted to do something significant and measurable to combat the growing problem of childhood obesity in this country, I'd do the following things to help turn the tide.

- I'd start the year off by testing my students in a number of different functional fitness activities, but I'd pay special attention to pull ups.

- I'd divide the students into two groups, those who can do at least one pull up (group X), and those who can't do any pull ups (group Y).

- I'd then divide the students up into teams of equal size, and each team would be required to have at least one student who can do a pull ups (from group X).

- I'd make the student(s) from group X responsible for helping students from group Y learn to do pull ups, and reward the successes accordingly.

- I'd create at least one (and probably three or four) height adjustable pull up station, and show all students how to use the strategy of leg assisted pull ups, "inching" their way up the chain until they eventually run out of leg assistance and can do regular pull ups.

- I'd also have a Total Gym to help students with extraordinary weight problems to make regular, measurable progress towards regular pull ups.

- I'd introduce a practical context within which kids would understand good nutritional habits, implement and monitor it.

- I'd make sure that everyone from group X knows how to work correctly with their teammates from group Y.

- I'd intentionally stack the deck and build small but regular successes (motivation) into the program for all participants

- I'd make quarterly checks to see what's happening in each group.

- I'd check out the possibility of having some intra-class, intra-grade, even intra-school competitions, being careful to compare group to group instead of individual student to individual student.

- As far as individual students are concerned, I'd encourage self-competition over competition with other students.

- The first goal is to make sure that all participants make regular, tangible progress over a significant period of time…at least 12 weeks. This will establish a pattern of public success, and internalize the motivation.

- The primary, long term goal of course would be to significantly increase the percentage of students who are members of group X from quarter to quarter, semester to semester, year to year.

- I'd generate regular press releases (on school letterhead) so the local media could be kept updated and would report regularly on how we're attacking childhood obesity in our school.

- I'd build a PYOW web-site so that the computerized generation can check out all kinds of related things whenever they're on line.

- I'd involve the private sector, many of whom are anxious to be identified with, even sponsor public educational success in a variety of ways.
- I'd organize an annual Pull Up A Thon between schools to help raise funds to benefit a worthwhile, local charity.

- I'd try to track all kinds of related behaviors, including academic success.

- I'd make it a privilege to participate. Forcing participation turns pull ups into a job and effectively reduces its value to students.

- I'd take advantage of the fact that all students want to be strong, not weak, and I'd cultivate a mentality favoring strength and independence over weakness and dependence.

- I'd tell other physical educators about this program and encourage them to develop programs of their own for their own students.

- I'd find companies in the area who'd like to sponsor PYOW employee wellness programs, and have students explain and design their program.

- I'd find police and fire departments who'd like to participate and have students explain and design their program.

- I'd find educators in schools who'd like to participate and have students explain and design their program.

- I'd find parents who'd like to participate and have students design their PYOW program.

- I'd go to city hall and recruit politicians who'd like to participate, etc.

- I'd go to park districts, Boy's and Girl's Clubs, YM/WCA's, Health Clubs, Pre-Schools, and churches, to find out who else in the community would like to be able to physically Pull Their Own Weight, then encourage the students to help them do so.

- I'd encourage students to take pride in their peer's, (and generally in other people's) success.

- And I'll add more things to do when and if they come to me.

PYOW: Criticisms & Obstacles

As simple and workable as PYOW seems to be, and with as much good publicity as it has received, it was never without its critics. So what kind of obstacles and criticisms has the program had to overcome in order to succeed? Here are the issues that most commonly came up.

It Lacks Hard, Scientific Evidence

Yes, that's true. Despite the fact that several exercise physiologists have agreed that it would be an interesting project, nobody that I know of has ever done a scientific study designed to reveal the body composition differences between kids who can and kids who can't do pull ups. That is to say, the only evidence I have is all the kids I observed with my own two eyes during almost two decades of teaching and coaching.

By the same token, nobody that I know of has ever done a scientific study designed to reveal whether your nose is on your face or not either. Perhaps both studies are too simple and intuitively obvious to interest academia.

Most Kids Hate Pull Ups

Yes, that's also true. Then again most kids hate to fail in public at anything...including reading, writing, and arithmetic. The trick is to start kds young, present PYOW in the right light (as a privilege instead of an obligation or a job), and to build public success into the program for every participant. Do these things and you'll be amazed how quickly kids learn to look forward to their chance to get on the pull-up bar. By the way, the same formula works for reading, writing, and arithmetic too.

It Lacks Comprehensiveness

As it turned out, the most common criticism came from people who felt that the program was too limited, that it was lacking in comprehensiveness, and therefore it failed to cover many important aspects of a good fitness program.

But in my view, these critics failed to understand that nobody ever claimed that PYOW was a comprehensive fitness program. It never pretended to be. *What you have here is a very simple and functional antidote to childhood obesity*. Its sole claim is that if you can do pull-ups, you cannot be obese. That's the golden rule of PYOW. Learn to do pull ups, maintain the ability, and you'll be a permanent member of Wall A, and never ever a member of Wall B again."

On the other hand, even though PYOW completely almost totally ignores the aerobic aspect of fitness (for example), to the degree that it discourages excess body weight, it also reduces the workload on the heart 24 hours a day, seven days a week, right? So you don't have to be a rocket scientist to see that PYOW is definitely heart friendly, right?

Skinny Kids Who Can't...

We had several people say, "There are plenty of skinny kids who can't do pull ups, so just because you can't do pull ups certainly doesn't mean you're obese." In short, these folks are absolutely correct in their observation.

On the other hand, obesity does exclude the ability to do pull ups. That is to say, show me a kid who's obese, and I'll show you a kid who can't do pull ups. Show me a kid who can do pull ups, and I'll show you a kid who's not obese. And finally, show me a kid who can do lots of pull ups, and I'll show you a kid who's lean.

PYOW Discourages Other Forms of Exercise

Furthermore, others felt that since PYOW's focus was pull-ups, that it discouraged other forms of exercise. But if these critics had taken a closer look, they'd find that *PYOW encourages anything that improves pull-up performance*, including other forms of exercise, which also burn calories, and help control or reduce the participant's body weight (their workload on the pull-up bar). It also recognizes the role of good eating habits, getting sufficient rest, and flexibility. Pull-ups however, are still the bottom line, functional acid test for PYOW.

PYOW Is Too Good To Be True

A similar criticism was that anything that simple cannot possibly work. In other words, if it looks too good to be true, it probably is too good to be true.

To that charge, I simply go back to the Wall A, Wall B example. As a matter of fact, I contended this criticism was picking on the program's greatest strength…its sheer simplicity, its financial and logistical accessibility.

So, What Exactly Is A Pull Up?

There was some debate over the question, what constitutes a pull up? There was a gym teacher involved in the conversation who originally contended that there should be "no kicking allowed, because that was cheating." I even had one young entrepreneurial lad suggest, *"If I can do ten pull ups half way up, that should count for five full pull ups…right Coach?"* But after talking it over, we decided to simplify the whole thing by saying that a participant had to go all the way down (straight arms), and all the way up (chin touching the bar), and anything in between was acceptable. In other words, when starting from the original down position, you'd be allowed to kick, twist, scream, or holler, in order to reach that final up position. Our mantra in this regard was "all the way down, and all the way up. Anything else goes." And that's exactly how we defined a pull up at Jefferson Elementary School back in the early 90's.

The Medical Community Recommends A More Complicated Solution

Let's have a look at the conventional, comprehensive, solution to the childhood obesity epidemic offered by experts from St. Louis Children's Hospital: Check it out.

1. Work together on one positive change at a time. You can set your child up for failure by trying to make too many changes as once.
2. Get rid of the junk food. Make fruits, vegetables and other healthy snacks readily available and eliminate junk food to avoid temptation.
3. Turn off the TV. Get rid of distractions during mealtime and concentrate on enjoying the food and spending time together.

4. Offer options to your child. Rigid guidelines can alter a child's internal sense of hunger and satiety. When offered options, a child learns to make positive choices consistently.
5. Beware of beverages. Juice and colas can add hundreds of calories a day.
6. Limit snacks and control portion sizes. It is unreasonable to give a child a bag of chips and expect him to stop after a few. Help your child out by putting a snack in a bowl ahead of time.
7. Give positive feedback. Take notice when your child makes steps toward changing bad habits, such ass choosing an apple for an after-school snack.
8. Limit "screen time." Encourage active pursuits by allowing only an hour a day for sedentary time with video games, the computer and the television.
9. Do it together. You don't have to plan a workout to get exercise. Family fun, such as playing in the sprinkler, diving into leaves or having snowball fights, burns calories, too.
10. Consider your child's feelings. Teaching you child healthy eating habits is a long-term goal,

but be sensitive about when to give it a rest and let him enjoy the things that children enjoy.

PYOW in contrast, says learn to perform pull-ups at an early age, do what ever it takes to maintain that wonderful ability for as long as you want to remain relatively strong and trim. Now, I ask which one is simpler? Which one is more tangible and measurable in terms of progress, and therefore motivation? Which one is easier to understand, afford and to implement? And if it's simpler, more measurable, more affordable, and more implementable, which approach has the best odds of succeeding? If you said PYOW, you win!

Other Exercises Can Make The Same Claims, So Why Just Pull Ups?

Another common criticism was that you can make the same claims for other activities such as dips, hand stand push ups, and say a seven minute mile. If you can do any of these things, you'll also be relatively lean and strong.

To that criticism I can only say…"I agree!" And again, we never discouraged students from doing other forms of exercise. The reason we settled on pull-ups was that everyone knows what they are. Where some people may not know what you mean by dips or hand-stand push-ups. And a seven-minute mile takes lots more space, good weather, and lots more time to develop.

But most importantly, *only pull-ups are associated with the phrase "Pull Your Own Weight."* And this phrase has many other positive connotations naturally built into it. So we settled on pull-ups instead of dips, hand stand push-ups, or seven-minute miles.

Boys Will Have An Advantage Over Girls

I've had an occasional feminist suggest that boys would have an advantage over girls in this testosterone-laden activity.

My response to this one was that "these critics never saw the girls at Jefferson school who, because they often mature faster than boys, were often the best pull-up performers in class. So this criticism was simply untrue."

PYOW Will Make Girls Masculine

Along the same line of thinking there were some who suspected that PYOW would make the little girls masculine, and give them bulging muscles.

Again, his answer was that these critics never saw the girls at Jefferson School. Factually speaking girls don't have the hormones to develop masculinity unless they take them (i.e., steroids) artificially. So, once again I simply say if they'd the girls at Jefferson School, they'd already know they're wrong!

PYOW Could Prove Embarrassing, And Further Alienate Real Heavy Kids

Another critic asked what about those kids who have gotten real heavy at a real young age? Won't OPYOW put them on the defensive, on the outside looking in, and feeling even worse about themselves than they already do?

In response, I simply don't remember any kids who failed to succeed if we lowered the bar enough to allow them to get their chin up and over the bar. And if you succeed regularly in public, there's very little to be embarrassed about. After several weeks of regular public success, the embarrassment issue was ancient history. We were also lucky enough to have two Total Gyms in house, and on that machine anybody can easily succeed immediately.

You Don't Need A Degree To Teach It, So What Good Can It Be?

I had one humorous (tongue in cheek) teacher say, "if you don't have to have a degree to teach it, how good can it be?"

Again, my response was that these critics were attacking PYOW's greatest strength—its simplicity. Actually many of the parents who became PYOW moms and dads *had no degrees at all. They were school dropouts.* But the changes that occurred in the kids they worked with, often rubbed off on the parents and put a wind in their sails that they'd never experienced before.

Many teachers noticed that parents got as much out of the program as the kids did. So one of its inadvertent strengths was its ability to generate parental involvement, enthusiasm, and even confidence, which, in at risk populations, is usually a hard nut to crack. Without ever planning to do so, PYOW became the primary parental involvement vehicle for the entire grant.

How About Liability Issues?

Another obstacle that came up at Jefferson School was this question of school liability. All school administrators these days run scared in the face of liability issues and lawsuits, so that's a legitimate concern.

I confess that in the school setting, every administration will have to make its own call. On the other hand, if leg assisted pull-ups were the most dangerous activity their students experience, they have almost no problems at all.

The other thought is that PYOW is certainly not restricted to schools. It can easily be done in YM/WCA's, Park Districts, Boys & Girls Clubs or Churches. For that matter PYOW can easily be done in the home by concerned parents. The equipment cost is negligible, the space required is minimal, and as we said before, you definitely don't need a degree to teach it!

What If There's No Mandate From The Top Down?

One other criticism has been that K-3 teachers at Jefferson School were mandated to participate, but in other schools, teachers may just choose to avoid participation. What then?

The fact of the matter is at Jefferson School teachers were mandated from top down to participate, and there were definitely teachers who resented it. They felt like they were overworked already (they probably were) and that PYOW was taking time from more important subjects like reading, writing and arithmetic. And nobody could argue that it didn't displace these other activities. But it was those same teachers who drug their feet, lacked enthusiasm, and shorted their kids in the process, and in my view, they should never be allowed to be a part of a PYOW program anyway.

And because of this issue, I recommend that PYOW should only be used by teachers who understand the concept, see the importance of it, and who will enthusiastically work with kids in the program. Furthermore, teachers who enthusiastically want to participate will be the exception, not the rule. Let the enthusiastic teachers light the fire and lead the way. Let them show their colleagues what can be achieved through an incredibly simple program.

Pull Your Own Weight Is Selfish

There were a couple people who interpreted the phrase Pull Your Own Weight as "selfish." That is to say, in a social context, they understood it to mean take care of yourself...ONLY, and forget about other people. But in my view they were missing the point. From a social standpoint the point was, "if you're unable to take care of your own affairs, the odds of you being in a position to help other people is worse than bad. On the other hand, people who learn to pull their own weight in all kinds of ways, are almost always in positions to teach others how to pull their weight, and in the process they will develop self respect as well as a healthy (as opposed to a condescending) respect for other people." This little "teach 'em to fish" recognition we called *Pull Your Own Weight Plus.*

PYOW Gets Too Much Good Publicity

The final criticism I'll mention is one that came from Dr. Peter Flynn who was the Superintendent of Davenport Public Schools back then. He complained to me one day "That PYOW program gets more good publicity than all the rest of the (20 school) district gets combined."

Another tongue in cheek criticism for sure, but my answer was simply, "If your school or your school district appreciates good ink, PYOW is hard to beat." That's pretty much the gamut as far as criticisms and obstacles, now let's talk about some other lifelong lessons that are packed in between the lines of Operation Pull Your Own Weight

A Simple, Home Made Childhood Obesity Prevention Machine That Really Works

Operation Pull Your Own Weight is a childhood obesity prevention strategy that's built on three simple observations, including:

1. **Kids who can do pull ups ARE NEVER OBESE**
2. If you start them young, and use leg assisted pull ups in conjunction with a height adjustable pull up bar, **ALMOST ALL KIDS can learn to do pull ups**.
3. As long as they maintain the ability to do pull ups, **almost all kids can NATURALLY IMMUNIZE THEMSELVES against obesity for a lifetime** without ever having to resort to pills, shots, or special diets to do the trick.

After hearing these observations, people often ask, "OK, so what are leg assisted pull ups? And what's a height adjustable pull up bar? And where can I buy one and help my kids to immunize themselves against obesity for a lifetime?"

Of LAPU's and HAPUB's...

First of all *leg assisted pull ups* are the ones that are done with the help of a participant's legs. In other words the participant is jumping and pulling at the same time in order to get their chin up to the bar.

A *height adjustable bar* accommodates leg assisted pull ups because it can be raised or lowered in one inch increments in order to increase or decrease the amount of leg assistance along with the level of difficulty individually for each performer. By raising the bar, the participant lowers the amount of leg assistance, and increases the level of difficulty.

The idea is to start at a height where the participant can do at least eight LAPU's, and gradually increase the repetitions to twelve. When the participant can do twelve LAPU's, *the bar is raised one inch*, and the entire eight to twelve scenario is repeated.

As the bar is gradually raised in one inch increments over time, the participant eventually runs out of leg assistance, and discovers that they're suddenly able to do conventional pull ups. That is to say, they can officially pull their own weight, and have now naturally immunized themselves against obesity for a lifetime, so long as they maintain their hard won ability.

So Where Can You Buy One?

So where can you buy a height adjustable pull up bar? Honestly, to my knowledge nobody is currently manufacturing a height adjustable pull up bar that raises and lowers in one inch increments. But that doesn't mean you can't make one yourself. The remainder of this article then is dedicated to explaining *how simple it is to make a home made height adjustable pull up bar. Check it out.*

Here Are The Ten Things You'll Need...

1. One doorway pull up bar to install permanently (preferably screwed in)
2. One roll of galvanized hanger strap, sometimes called plumber's tape
3. Two, three foot sections of chain with one inch links
4. Two Quick Links (Home Depot's terms...an oval shaped link with a screw based opening and closing connecting mechanism)
5. Two eye bolts
6. Two Spring Links (Home Depot terms...a tear drop shaped, spring loaded connecting mechanism)
7. One pipe, one inch in diameter that's six inches wider than your doorway

8. Two rubber floor protectors. These are normally used on the bottoms of chairs to protect the floor, but in this case you place on each end of the pipe.
9. One wooden ruler, three feet long
10. One drill, one screwdriver, and one crescent wrench*

Sixteen Simple Steps

With these components in hand, *follow 16 simple steps* and you'll have your very own, cost effective, home made, childhood obesity prevention machine (a.k.a. a height adjustable pull up bar) with which *your kids can teach themselves* how to do pull ups, and in the process they can immunize themselves against obesity for the rest of their lives as long as they maintain their ability to perform pull ups.

1. Permanently install the doorway pull up bar, preferably using screws
2. Mount the wooden ruler vertically along the side of the doorway
3. Cut two lengths of plumber's tape long enough overlap by two inches when wrapped completely around the pipe

4. Saddle these over the pull up bar attach the Quick Links to each one
5. Attach one section of chain to each Quick Link so that they hang from the bar
6. Close both Quick Links tightly
7. Drill a hole (two holes) about two inches *from each end of the pipe*
8. Insert the eye bolts into the holes and secure tightly with accompanying nut
9. Attach one teardrop shaped Spring Link into each eye bolt
10. With the Spring Links, attach your pull up bar horizontally to any pair of chain links and record the height by referring to the ruler mounted in the doorway
11. Now using your legs to jump and your arms to pull simultaneously do at least eight leg assisted pull ups.
12. If you can't do eight repetitions, lower the bar until you can do eight reps
13. Your next workout you'll do nine, then ten, then eleven, then twelve reps
14. When you can do twelve repetitions, raise the bar one inch and begin the entire eight to twelve rep scenario all over again

15. As you make regular progress workout after workout, week after week, the bar will get so high that you'll eventually run out of legs and be real doing pull ups.
16. Maintain that ability for the rest of your life and you'll always be relatively strong and relatively trim...and NEVER OBESE.

The Recipe for Success...

Now that you have access to the equipment, the recipe for success includes...

1. Regular workouts, twice a week, on non-consecutive days
2. Eat a well balanced diet including plenty of fruits and veggies
3. Get sufficient rest at night
4. Avoid tobacco, it makes you weak
5. Avoid alcohol, it makes you weak
6. Avoid drugs, they make you weak
7. And get stronger almost every time you work out

Questions?

If you have further questions check out the official *Operation Pull Your Own Weight web site* at www.pullyourownweight.net or the blog entitled www.childhood-obesity-prevention.com. They're both loaded with good, practical information designed for good, practical parents who want to do something to prevent their kids from childhood obesity and all the problems that go along with it.

*Make sure that all these components **are strong enough to hold MORE** than the weight of the children (or the adults) who will be using it.

Lifelong Lessons That Are Packed In Between The Lines Of OPYOW...

After four years working with elementary school age kids we found that although our focus was on improving self esteem by avoiding obesity, there was lots more learning going on than what we'd originally expected. I had many a teacher tell me that there were lessons hidden between the lines of PYOW, and that they were almost as important as the main lesson we were aiming to teach. So without further adieu, let's have a quick look at some of those lessons.

The Significance of Self Esteem

There are lots of things that can be said about PYOW and education generally speaking, starting with self esteem. For example, to the degree that a higher level of physical fitness improves a student's confidence (self-esteem) in his/her ability to try something new and succeed, it has a global effect on almost everything he/she does from the social to the academic arena. On the other hand kids who lack confidence (self-esteem) are often afraid to try new things. As the result, they effectively prevent themselves from growing and learning. And that's pretty big thing to learn at an early age.

But in digging a little deeper on this question, one of the most interesting things that I learned was that PYOW makes a wonderful *'advance organizer.'* If that's an unfamiliar term to you, don't feel like the Lone Ranger. Look it up on the internet and you'll find numerous references that are informative and insightful. But the following paragraph is representative of what you'll discover.

A Mental Scaffolding Upon Which To Grow

"David Ausubel is a psychologist who advanced a theory which contrasted meaningful learning from rote learning. In Ausubel's view, to learn meaningful, students must relate new knowledge (concepts and propositions) to what they already know. He proposed the notion of an advanced organizer as a way to help students lik their ideas with new material or concepts. Ausubel's theory of learning claims that new concepts to be learned can be incorporated into more inclusive concepts or ideas. These more inclusive concepts or ideas are advance organizers. Advance organizers can be verbal phrases (the paragraph you are about to read is about Albert Einstein), or a graphic. "

In any case, the advance organizer is designed to provide, what cognitive psychologists call, the "mental scaffolding: to learn new information. Ausubel believed that learning proceeds in a top-down, or deductive manner. Ausubel's theory consists of three phases, presentation of an advance organizer, presentation of learning task or material, and strengthening the cognitive organization."

PYOW As An Advance Organizer

So, how does PYOW serve as a mental scaffolding upon which to construct new and meaningful knowledge? Check this out. Kids who are participating in a PYOW program are learning the following lessons in a very tangible, and hands-on way.

First, the teacher sets the PYOW stage by reading the kids a story, which you saw previously. As you'll recall, the story is basically a conversation between a kindergartner named Johnny and his high school age cousin Jamal. Johnny wants to grow up to be strong and cool like Jamal. So in the story Johnny is faced with the choice between becoming strong and fit like Jamal, or weak, and unfit (even fat, obese) which is definitely uncool for Johnny, and all kids who hear the story.

Strong VS Weak...A Language That Motivates Kids...

Now everyone associates exercise with getting strong and fit. So when the teacher introduces the pull up bar, the kids readily accept that doing pull-ups will help make them strong. *And again, all kids, boys and girls alike, want to be strong, and none of them want to be weak.* They also want to be fit and lean (it's cool), not overweight (that's uncool), so all this naturally works its way into the whole PYOW conversation.

The interesting thing is that once the concepts of strong and weak are introduced and ingrained on the pull-up bar, they can easily be carried over into many other aspects of a child's life, including a their academic work. In other words, do you want to be strong or weak in math, science, English, and history? Any teacher who chooses to do so can use the context of strong VS weak to frame many other areas of student growth, and win over all those kids who want to be bad, *but certainly don't want to be weak in any way.*

Pull Ups: A Privilege, Not An Obligation

Pull Your Own Weight was always presented as something that students get to do, not something they have to do. That is to say, nobody forced them to participate. They chose to participate of their own free will. It was lots like going to a Bears, Bulls, Cubs, or Sox game, or going to see your favorite rock star, or a movie that you want to see.

These are all privileges, and as such they are valued in a way that an obligation (or a job) is not valued. Kids pick up on this quickly. If professional educators would present education generally speaking as a privilege instead of an obligation (a job starting at age five), they'd be much more successful in achieving their goals, and they'd accomplish them with much less hassle. After all, presented right, education should be a privilege.

Setting Goals, Working Regularly, Producing Progress, Leads To Success

Participants learn that when they set a realistic, concrete goal (like being able to perform pull ups), and work consistently towards it, over a period of time (persistence), they will produce regular progress, which adds up to lots of progress over time, and eventually allows them to reach their end goal.

Now the same holds true for anything else you want to learn whether it's math or science, the piano, basketball, or Tai Kwon Do. If you set your goal, work regularly, and expect to make regular progress towards that goal, your odds of eventually reaching your destination increase dramatically.

Thin Slices Of Progress Over Time Add Up To Large Chunks Of Success

Furthermore they learn that the improvement occurs in very small increments, or as we called them...slices of progress. In the case of PYOW you're improving by one repetition, or moving one inch higher each workout. And if you pile all those thin slices of improvement on top of one another, they eventually add up to large chunks of improvement. Now wouldn't you agree that the same things are true of anything else that you want to learn, improve, or get stronger in? Yes, what we're really talking about here is persistence.

Eating Right & Getting Enough Rest Makes You Strong

Let's keep going here. In the PYOW experience a student also learns that eating right, and getting sufficient rest pays off in strength gain on the pull-up bar. Again, this is a lesson that can be carried over into every other subject in life, whether inside or outside of school?

But Tobacco, Alcohol, And Drugs Make You Weak

And finally, they also learn that negative habits like tobacco, alcohol, and drugs, make you weak on the pull-up bar, just like they make you weak in almost every other aspect of life. And yes, even so called strength enhancement drugs like steroids, eventually tear you down and make you weak in the long run.

The Responsibility Is All Yours, Nobody Else Can Do It For You, But It Sure Helps When They Cheer You On!

And maybe the most essential lesson learned in this simple solution to a complicated problem, is the fact that the child must do the work, and persist through to the end...themselves. In other words nobody else can do the work for them. If they want to get strong, develop a functional antidote to obesity, and learn all the other lessons contained in PYOW, then it's up to them to earn it. And for my money, this lesson goes a long ways in this day and age of people blaming others for things that they could have taken care of themselves, if they'd just developed the strength and know how to pull their own weight.

So How Does PYOW Effect A Child's Education?

So when someone wants to know how PYOW affects the general educational experiences of a participant, let's recognize that confidence gained from anything including physical fitness increases the odds of succeeding in almost anything. And if you have it built into your experiential Rolodex that setting goals, working regularly, and persistently generating results in thin slices

189

of improvement that pile up over time, and grow into large chunks of improvement and success, you're on the right track.

If they learn early that good eating and sufficient rest plays a positive role in their strength development, and if they know that tobacco, alcohol and drugs makes them weak, the choice for most kids will be strong, not weak. Now I'd say by itself that's a pretty good foundation for an education. What do you think?

PYOW As The Main Job Of Education

If PYOW represents a hands-on reference, a mental-scaffolding on which to build new and meaningful knowledge, wouldn't you agree that the odds of a kid succeeding are enhanced dramatically by participation? Don't you agree that we should teach as many kids as we can to move over onto Wall A, and away from Wall B, to pull their own weight, to set goals, to take the responsibility, to work regularly toward achieving them, and that this approach will result in the successful achievement of their goals? In the end isn't the goal of education to teach kids how to pull their own weight in all kinds of ways? If you agree, I say, let's get after it today.

PYOW In Police and Fire Departments, Education, the Military, Corporate Wellness, and Congress

Although PYOW is a program designed primarily for kids who want to avoid all the problems related to childhood obesity, that doesn't mean that its principals don't carry over well into adulthood, so long as the participant stays on Wall A by maintaining their ability to perform pull ups. But I do have people ask, what about older kids and adults? Doesn't PYOW work for them?

The obvious answer is that since we're advocating in continuance for as long as you want to avoid becoming overweight, the gold rule of PYOW – people who can do pull ups cannot be obese, and people who are obese cannot do pull ups - holds true regardless of age or gender. It just doesn't matter.

I'm also regularly asked if adults can use the same simple height adjustable pull up bar/leg assisted pull ups technique that kindergartners use so successfully?   And I reply, that technique will work for anyone who wants to dedicate themselves to learning to perform this simple exercise. I will admit however that it's easier for a kindergartner, before they've gained weight than it is for the older teenager or the adult who has picked up unwanted pounds. But in either case, persistence is the key, and persistence will win out.

Now of special interest to me in our adult population are the men and women who make up our nation's police force, our fire departments, our military, and our nation's teachers. Let's check these out one at a time.

Police Officers

How many times have you seen an overweight police officer carrying a cup of coffee and a box of Krispee Kreams out of a donut shop and asked yourself, "How is this guy going to catch up with bad guys in the street, or protect me and my family from anything, ever? Are we not paying these folks to at least be physically competent?" On the other hand, policemen are human and they're subject to the same temptations that are bloating the bellies and lining the veins and arteries of our entire high tech, fast food oriented culture, right?

So who's to blame, the cop or the system who tempts him? Yep, cops can get fat just like the rest of us, so what can we do about the problem. On the other hand I guarantee that there are precious few police officers who would be unable to learn to do pull ups if they put their minds to the task. Not only that, but I promise that every police officer who can do pull ups will not be obese...just like any kid. It just can't happen, it's just that simple.

Fire Departments

How about the men and women who make up our nation's fire departments? These people have lots of time to sit around, read, and watch the boob tube when they're not in action. But when they're in action, there's little time for thinking and little sympathy for someone who moves too slow because they're lugging around excess weight. After all in this occupation, the stakes are life and death all the time.

Now these days most fire houses are equipped with workout rooms including weights, plates, treadmills, and steppers. And the percentage of overweight firemen is probably very low in comparison to the other two groups we're looking at here. But again, they are human which means they are tempted when they drive past McDonald's or Baskin Robbins on their way to and from work. There are also a similar percentage who have slow metabolisms to contend with, so they have to battle the weight problem just like the rest of us do.

However, since they generally have the time and the facility, teaching fire department members would be relatively easy. And I would reiterate that members who can do pull ups can't be obese, and if there's such a thing as an overweight fireman, he will be unable to perform pull ups.

Educators

Let's move on to teachers now. Teachers are often people who young people generally look up to, especially in their early years and when teachers are obese, it delivers the wrong kind of message to impressionable kids. And the worst of these is the proverbial overweight gym teacher, male or female, who preaches fitness in class, but who obviously falls far short of the mark himself.

But let me assure you that it doesn't matter if you're a gym teacher or a music teacher, a science teacher, or an art teacher – any teachers who can do pull ups can't be obese, and any teachers who are obese can't do pull ups, I guarantee it. And like the police and fire department members we mentioned previously, there are very few teachers who are unable to learn to perform pull ups once they decide they want to do it. So yes, I'm in favor of teaching teachers to physically pull their own weight.

Corporate Wellness

Is Health Care a major issue for corporate America today? Is the Pope Catholic? Now can you imagine a simpler, time efficient, more implementable corporate wellness program than teaching all employees to physically pull their own weight? It eliminates obesity and all the related problems. Instead it generates strength, improves self esteem and it magnifies all the good the good things that go along with that. How about it Mr. CEO, how'd you like to have employees who can pull their own weight physically, and in all kinds of other ways as well? Do you think that'd alleviate some of your health care issues?

The Military and Congress

Finally there are the men and women who make up our armed forces. Like the firemen, there's down time in the military, but when the buzzer goes off, they must be physically and mentally ready to take action. And by simply teaching them all to pull their own weight and to maintain the ability, they will beat the growing tendency in this country to become overweight...even in the military. My final thought is Congress. As long as we're looking for a challenge, Henry Hyde I want to teach you to do pull ups!

The Operation PYOW

Appendix

Dr. Tommy Boone Has Been Pulling His Own Weight For Some Time Now

When Tommy Boone was eight years old his dad installed a pull-up bar in the doorway of the bedroom he shared with his brother. For a full year afterwards, Mr. Boone encouraged his sons to develop the ability to do more and more pull-ups. "But after the first year," Tommy said, "pull-ups became a regular habit for both of us. Every time we walked into the bedroom, and every time we walked out, we did a couple of pull-ups, and to this day I'm still relatively strong for my age."

Pull-ups Translate Into Long Term Fitness

The pull-up habit that Mr. Boone instilled into his sons helped the boys develop more and more upper body strength, and related sporting interests as they grew into adulthood. "In my case," Tommy said, "the pull-up bar translated into an interest in gymnastics, which in turn led me to Northwestern Louisiana State University where I competed as a gymnast for four years while majoring in Physical Education." To be even more accurate, Tommy Boone was *an All American Gymnast* in 1966, and the pull-up bar his dad installed when he was eight served as a guiding light.

Dad Was An Attorney, But...

Occupationally speaking, Boone's father was an attorney as well as a State Senator who worked with legendary populist icon Huey (the Kingfish) Long who cast a lengthy shadow in Louisiana politics. "My dad always wanted me to go to law school and follow in his footsteps, so he was a little disappointed when I first announced my intention to study Physical Education and to coach," Boone said.

"On the other hand," he continued, "my dad was always keenly aware of, and sensitive to the importance of physical strength and health, and the doorway pull-up bar is a great indicator of that recognition. In any case, after a couple of years into my studies at Northwestern, Dad pulled me aside one day and confessed that he'd reconsidered, and thought I may be onto something interesting after all."

From an Undergrad to a Ph.D.

As it turned out, Mr. Boone's speculative insight turned out to be prophetic as fitness developed into a full-fledged industry in the seventies and eighties. Tommy followed his own teaching and coaching dreams, by finishing up his Masters at Northwestern, and promptly took a teaching and coaching position at Northeast Louisiana State University, in Monroe, LA, in 1968, then, acquired a teaching position at the University of Florida in 1969. He stayed for two years, but despite being encouraged to hang on to the job, Boone transferred to Florida State University to pursue a Ph.D. in Exercise Physiology.

Leapfrogging Into the Future

Leapfrogging into the future, Dr. Tommy Boone has covered lots of ground since those Florida days. Currently, he Chairs the Department of Exercise Physiology at The St. Scholastica College in Duluth, MN where he has been since 1993-94. He has also been published so many times (articles, books, web sites, blogs, etc.) that he could single handedly prevent an entire Department from perishing if he really wanted to.

The American Society of Exercise Physiologists

He's also the co-founder and the first President of the *American Society of Exercise Physiologists* (the ASEP) an international group of over 500 Exercise Physiologists who are dedicated to rescuing related research from the ivory tower, and translating it into hands-on practicality in order to be implemented by real people, in real families, who reside on real streets in real neighborhoods around the real world.

Boone Warns Against the Dangers of Groupthink...

In an insightful essay entitled *Too Much Groupthink Leads to Conformity and Failure,* Boone chronicled eight deadly sins of groupthink including mindguarding, stereotyping, self-censorship, rationalization, direct pressure, the illusion of unanimity, the illusion of morality, and the illusion of invulnerability; *all of which work against the odds of finding real solutions to real problems (i.e., childhood obesity) in today's world.* Groupthink can be a major obstacle to creative problem solving when hierarchies, budgets, and individuals who are all being paid to think conventionally, come together and actively avoid getting to far out of their own respective comfort zones.

Comfort Zones Need Not Apply

In Boone's own words, "The ASEP *is not an organization for researchers who want to stay in their own comfort zone.* Exercise Physiology in our eyes, is all about improving quality of life for people around the world. If we fail to accomplish that, we're missing our target." So hands on practicality is a quality that's woven deep into the bones of Dr. Tommy Boone, and odds are all that was given a major league jump start back when his dad installed a simple doorway pull-up bar, and encouraged his sons to learn the hands on lessons of value created by regular work over a period of time.

Practical Advice for Today's Parents

Speaking of bringing the research down to street level, we decided to ask Dr. Tommy Boone what kind of advice he could offer 21st century parents who are wrestling with the issues such as childhood obesity and fitness in the face of TV, video games, computers, cars taking them everywhere, and Physical Education curriculums being cut faster than you can say No Child Left Behind? He offered the following advice.

"The most important thing parents can ever do for kids is to model the things that you want them to do. Actions always speak louder than words," Boone said. "If you want your kids to eat right, show them how by eating right yourself. If you want them to be physically active then you'd better be ready to walk the walk…literally. If you want them to avoid tobacco, alcohol and drugs, then set the right example yourself. If you say one thing and do another, you'll lose all your credibility. And when parents lack credibility, we all lose. It's about that simple," he added.

The PYOW (Strong/Weak) Test

1. All kids want to be…
   a. Strong
   b. Weak

2. No kids want to be…
   a. Weak
   b. Strong

3. Doing pull ups helps to make you…
   a. Strong
   b. Weak

4. When doing pull ups it helps to be…
   a. Heavy
   b. Light

5. The more pull ups you can do…
   a. The stronger and lighter you must be
   b. The heavier and weaker you must be

6. If you want to learn to Pull Your Own Weight (do pull ups) it helps to…
   a. Practice regularly
   b. Eat better
   c. Do plenty of walking or running to burn off excess calories
   d. Get enough sleep at night
   e. Avoid using tobacco, alcohol, and drugs
   f. All of the above
   g. None of the above

7. When learning to do pull ups...
    a. It helps if someone else does the pull ups for you
    b. You have to do the work yourself...nobody else can do it for you

8. As long as you maintain your ability to perform pull ups...
    a. You'll never be obese, and you'll always be relatively strong
    b. You'll always be obese, and you'll never be strong

9. The habits that make you strong on the pull up bar...
    a. Make you strong in all kinds of other ways, including academics
    b. Make you weak in all kinds of ways, including academics

10. If you fail to make progress on the pull up bar...
    a. It's the teacher's fault
    b. It's your parent's fault
    c. It's your friend's fault
    d. Take responsibility for yourself and failure will be a thing of the past

11. If you're too much overweight
    a. You will be unable to do even one pull up
    b. You must be a girl

12. If you can do at least one pull up...
    a. You can't be much overweight
    b. You can't be a boy

13. If you can do lots of pull ups...
    a. You have to be pretty lean/slim
    b. You have to be a girl

14. Using tobacco makes you...
    a. Weak
    b. Strong

15. Using alcohol makes you...
    a. Strong
    b. Weak

16. Using drugs makes you...
    a. Weak
    b. Strong

17. Eating poorly makes you...
    a. Strong
    b. Weak

18. Allowing someone else to do your homework makes you...
    a. Strong
    b. Weak

19. Getting too little sleep at night makes you...
    a. Weak
    b. Strong

20. The simplest way to make sure that you never become overweight is...
    a. Learn, and always maintain the ability to do pull ups
    b. Wait until a big pharmaceutical company creates a magic pill
    c. Buy a piece of exercise equipment from a TV infomercial
    d. Learn, and always maintain the ability to do pull ups
    e. A and D

Pablo: The Little Boy Who Didn't Know He Couldn't...Yet

When Pablo came into this world he had one big advantage, which was that *he hadn't yet learned that he couldn't do certain things*. As the result he tried doing all kinds of things and he discovered, much to his amusement, that some of the things he tried he could do, while others he couldn't do...yet.

For example, he discovered that if he wanted to do so, he could stretch his arms, his legs, his fingers, and his toes out so they felt longer, or he could pull them back in so they felt shorter. He found that if he reached out and touched things he could find out what they felt like, hard, soft, cool, warm, smooth, rough, etc. He also found that if he could wrap his fingers and thumb around an object that he could kind of control it and bring it in closer. He could throw it on the floor, which is when he discovered that he could expect Mom and Dad to fetch and bring it back to him...a couple of times anyway.

He tried laying on his stomach, and rolling over to his back. Mom sat him up and he found that to be an interesting experience. He watched Mom and Dad do the things that they could do and Pablo wondered if he could do them too? The most interesting thing they did was to stand on their feet and legs, balance, and move around wherever they wanted to go. Mom helped Pablo to hang on to the high chair to help him to stand up and that worked out pretty good. But when he let go and tried to move across the room like Mom and Dad, Pablo fell right on his face. Dad picked him up, dusted Pablo off, and consoled him.

Mom And Dad Encouraged Pablo

But Mom and Dad kept encouraging Pablo to walk, the falls became easier, and one day several weeks after he began trying, he took his first four steps…and then he fell again. But four steps, that was something to celebrate, at least his Mom and Dad thought so. They kept encouraging him and Pablo kept walking and doing all kinds of new things all the time. Mom and Dad thought Pablo must be a very bright boy. And one of the other things Pablo learned was that if you keep trying to do the thing you want to do, the odds of doing it become better and better until you succeed.

In fact during his first four years of life, Pablo tried and learned to do all kinds of things all because he didn't yet know that he couldn't do them. And if he didn't know that he couldn't, then maybe he could. Not only that, but the only way Pablo could find out whether he could or couldn't do something, was to try it. That way he knew for sure. In other words, if he didn't try something, he'd never find out what he could do and what he couldn't do. It was about that simple. And Pablo wanted to know. For all these reasons Mom and Dad always thought that Pablo must be a very bright young boy.

Then Pablo Turned Five And Went To Kindergarten

Then when he turned five years old, Mom and Dad enrolled Pablo in kindergarten along with lots of other five year olds, and instead of comparing what he could do yesterday to what he could do today or tomorrow, the teacher taught Pablo to compare himself to the other kids in class. The teacher was very good at this kind of thing and she saw all kinds of things like some kids were tall and some were short, some had blonde hair and some had brunette hair, some were skinny and some were stocky, some were fast runners and some were slow runners. And most importantly to the teacher, there were some kids who were smart, some who were average, and some who were below average and she placed them all in groups that reflected this assessment of them.

Pablo Was Labeled Average

As it turned out the teacher put Pablo in the middle group, but he had no idea why. Anyway he learned this new way of looking at himself from the teacher. Then he found out that when he tried stuff because he didn't know that he couldn't, the way he'd always done, some of the kids would laugh and make fun of him if he failed to do what he was trying to do. They thought less of him when he tried and failed, and the teacher seemed to think less of him too.

From this experience Pablo learned that it was embarrassing and painful to fail in front of the other kids and he never knew that before. But once he learned that lesson, he decided to avoid trying when other people were around and in doing so, Pablo would avoid having the other kids make fun of him, laugh at him, and make him think less and less of himself.

Pablo Learned To Stop Trying

By the time his kindergarten year was over, Pablo had switched gears when it came to trying new things. Prior to kindergarten, as you will recall, Pablo didn't know that he couldn't, so he would try it and find out whether he could or not. And back then when he failed nobody made fun of him, his Mom and Dad encouraged him to keep trying, and so he'd persist until he learned how to walk, how to talk, and how to do all kinds of very difficult things, because he just kept going until he finally learned to do what he wanted to learn to do.

But once in school Pablo learned that failing in front of the teacher and the other kids was embarrassing, painful, and that the simple solution was to stop trying in front of them. At least then he had an excuse. After all…he wasn't trying, right? And when he stopped trying, he could no longer find out if he could or he couldn't do things. But at least he wasn't embarrassed, at least the other kids weren't laughing at him and making him feel bad about himself, because they wouldn't know if he could or couldn't because he refused to try.

Pablo Learns To Shoot Himself In The Foot

Now the problem that developed over time was the more that Pablo refused to try, the less he learned about what he could and could not do. And the less he learned, the more his teachers and his peers just presumed that he couldn't learn to do new things, otherwise he would. Nobody wants to be labeled a dummy.

By the time he'd reached junior high school Pablo was no longer in the middle group, he had been labeled a slow learner, and a low performer. Even Mom and Dad threw their hands up and bought into what the teachers said about Pablo. Apparently he was not bright like they'd originally thought. After all, all parents think their own kids are bright, but some of them have to be wrong, right?

Pablo Even Began To Believe His Teachers

Worst of all Pablo began to believe what the teachers and his peers said about him. He began to feel angry and frustrated when he was in school...which by now, he absolutely hated. He began getting in fights with other kids and giving teaches a hard time, so now he was also being labeled a behavior problem too. Pablo finally dropped out of school without graduating, without a high school diploma, and then he went looking for work.

He applied for job after job, but found that the market for young people who'd dropped out of school, and who were also considered behavior problems, was pretty bad. And the jobs he was offered paid so little that they guaranteed Pablo would stay on the bottom of the heap, no matter how hard he now tried.

Let's Go Over How All This Happened...

Now you can use your imagination and finish this story any way you'd like, but the main thing to understand is that Pablo, like almost every other kid who comes into this world, was born with a gift of curiosity which he turned into knowledge of many amazing things. He knew he didn't know that he couldn't do something unless he tried it and failed. Then he discovered that if he kept trying, sooner or later he'd often succeed.

So Pablo explored his environment, watched Mom and Dad, and he tried to do the things that he saw them doing. And this entire time Mom and Dad always encouraged and even expected him to be able to learn and do all these wonderful things, if he persisted, which he usually did.

But when he was enrolled in school with a teacher and with other kids, they taught him that if he tried and failed, that they'd make fun of him, and think less of him. And in the long run, they convinced Pablo that he couldn't do much of anything, and that it was no longer worth trying.

Pablo learned to hate school, his peers, and eventually to hate himself, all because he was systematically taught that he couldn't do things, and for whatever reason, he and his parents thought the school system knew what it professed to know. After all, these people have college degrees and they are smart, right? But once Pablo himself bought into their suggestion that he couldn't...his fate was sealed.

The First Really Good Question

Now, the first real question at this point is…who's to blame? How would you answer this controversial question?

- Is it the overworked and underpaid teacher who's given the task of sorting out the strengths and weaknesses of 25 to 30 kids each year in order to begin the selection and labeling process that we now call "education" in the 21st century?
- Is it the school administrators who are hired to oversee and operate the system?
- Is it local school board members who are elected to oversee and direct the administrators, and the school system?
- Is it the country, state, and federal educational administrators who concern themselves with marketing unfunded mandates like *No Child Left Behind*.
- Or is it Pablo's parents who presumed that the system knew what they were doing when it came to educating Pablo?
- Or Pablo himself who should have been stronger
- His peers who should have been more compassionate and understanding

- Or do each one of these parts kind of go along with the others while under the hypnotic presumption that questioning the system that's served this nation well so for over 200 years, is a sign of disrespect, disloyalty, is unpatriotic, and cannot be tolerated?
- And if you choose this last one, then who's in charge of evaluating the doggone system and what it's producing?

The Second Really Good Question

The second real question is, what can we do about this problem? What would you tell Pablo, his peers, his parents, his teachers, his school administrators, the school board who oversees the system? I know what I'd tell them. I'd say it's the expressed goal of this school system to teach Pablo and all his peers that the only way to find out if you can or you can't do something is to try doing it. And just because you can't do it today doesn't mean that you'll be unable to do it tomorrow…so long as you keep on trying. No, there really is no substitute for persistence.

I would say that in order to succeed the system must convince Pablo and his peers that there is absolutely nothing wrong with failing to perform, and there is everything wrong with failing to try. After all, in the big picture, human life is all about exploring and testing our

213

limits from day to day, plotting and planning how to push those limits back over weeks, months, and years.

Winning And Losing In Education

To the degree we achieve that goal, the system and everyone in it wins. To the degree we fail, everyone loses. As the old saying goes, a chain is only as strong as its weakest link. So the job of educational systems around the country is to do everything possible to produce strong links who know that if they only persist, they can probably learn to do whatever they really need to do.

It's the job of school systems to strengthen each and every one of those links, every day, every week, every month, and every year, and to make sure Pablo knows that if he keeps on trying, there's very little that he can't accomplish. On the other hand, when you give up on yourself and stop trying, you are limiting yourself, you are shooting yourself in the foot, and you are dooming yourself to failure in the future.

For me this is the biggest lesson a child can learn during their formative years, and it is what education in the best sense, is all about. Now how do we go about achieving that goal? We can start by checking out Johnny and Jamal in the next story.

Pull Your Own Weight: A Really Strong Story For Kids

Johnny was a kindergartner. But his cousin Jamal was a senior in high school and a star running back on the football team. Johnny always looked up to Jamal and hoped one day that he too would be a star athlete, with his picture in the newspaper, and people talking about him on television. Everyone thought Jamal was really cool.

One day after supper Jamal and Johnny were wrestling around on the living room floor. When the action slowed down and they were each catching their breath, Johnny said. "I want to be just like you when I grow up Jamal. Do you think I will be?"

Jamal thought for a moment before he answered. Finally he said "Johnny, if you really want to be strong like me *it's up to you*! If you play your cards right, you'll be strong in all kinds of ways. And if you play your cards wrong, you'll probably be weak. Now which would you rather be Johnny, weak or strong?

Johnny just smiled and said "I want to be strong just like you Jamal. But I don't understand what you mean about the cards. What do you mean when you say I have to play my cards right?

Set A Goal, Practice Regularly, & Get Strong

"Ok Johnny" let me give you an example of what I'm talking about so you'll understand. One way to get strong is by setting a goal and doing exercises, like for example…pull ups, right? Now I have lots of friends in my school who hate pull ups, but it's because they're weak, they weigh too much, and they can't do pull ups. So when the coach puts them on the pull up bar and they can't do anything but hang, they get totally embarrassed."

"But personally, I love pull ups because I'm strong, light, and I can do lots of 'em. You could say I'm a star on the pull up bar" said Jamal with a cool smile.

"But one of the reasons I'm strong and light is that I've practiced doing pull ups twice a week ever since I was in fifth grade when I decided that I wanted to be able to do more than anyone else in my class…which I did, because _I was the only one_ who practiced doing them."

"Now, seven years later, after I've made little slices of progress every week, every month, every year, I look back and see that all those little slices of progress have added up to a great big pile of progress, especially if you compare me to others who never practiced pull ups."

"Lots of my fellow students think I'm just a natural. What they don't know is that anyone can be really strong on the pull up bar if they just practice regularly over a long period of time. It's that simple."

"So" Johnny said, "if I practice regularly, I'll get strong like you, right Jamal?

You Gotta Eat Right

"Well that's the first and most important part of the strength recipe," replied Jamal. "But there are three more things that we need to talk about here Johnny. First we need to talk about the things you eat. That's really important too."

"For example if you eat lots of junk food like chips, soda pop, fries, and candy you'll be depriving your body of the nutrition it needs to get really strong. Not only that, junk food tends to make you overweight, even fat. And the more you weigh, the harder it is to pull your own weight…to do pull ups. So it's really important that you eat the right foods if you really want to get strong. Understand Johnny?"

"Yah, I understand Jamal," said Johnny. "So I should practice doing pull ups every week, eat right, and I'll get strong just like you, right Jamal?

You Gotta Get Your Rest

"Hang on Johnny. There are still two more things we need to talk about. The next one is getting your rest. You see as important as regular practice, and good eating habits are, it's also really important to get enough rest if you really want to get strong. See your body needs time to recover from work, that's why you only practice pull-ups twice a week…three times at the most. If you do more than that you won't recover enough to get really strong."

"Not only that, but you have to get to bed at night in order to get enough sleep. Lots of kids try to stay up too late, and get up too early, and their bodies don't get enough rest. They can't build the muscles necessary to be strong. Got it?"

"Got it Jamal. But you said there's one more thing, right? What is that?

And You Gotta Avoid Tobacco, Alcohol, and Drugs

"The last thing you need to know is that, even though lots of kids today think they're cool, things like cigarettes, alcohol, and drugs make you weak. The fact is that anybody can smoke cigarettes, drink alcohol, and do drugs. That doesn't take any talent."

"But the kids that I know who are into that stuff, just get weaker, and weaker. In other words those kids can't pull their own weight in any way. Not only that, they're afraid to try for fear of failing, just like those kids who are embarrassed by being on the pull up bar. Their fear causes them to escape and to become weak in all kinds of ways."

But if you practice regularly over a long period of time, eat right, get your rest, and stay away from things that make you weak, *you will be a star at almost everything you do Johnny.*"

You Mean I'll Be Good At Everything?

"I'll be good at everything? Will getting strong on the pull up bar make me better in other stuff too Jamal?"

"Good question Johnny" Jamal replied. And the answer is that the same habits that make you strong on the pull up bar like regular practice, good eating, and getting enough rest, will help make you strong at anything else that you really want to do. You just have to decide what's important, practice regularly, eat right, get enough rest, and over time you'll see those thin slices of progress piling up into big chunks of progress that will make you strong in all those things that you choose to do. And that's called pulling your own weight in all kinds ways" he added.

"So now do you understand what I said about playing your cards, right Johnny? And do you understand that whether you become strong or weak is pretty much up to you? And do you also understand that it's up to you to choose those things that'll make you strong, and avoid those things that'll make you weak.

The better you are at making those choices Johnny, the stronger you'll be. Right?

"Got it" said Johnny with a great big smile.

"Now" Jamal said "let me show you how to work out on that pull up bar and you'll be pulling your own weight before you know it."

THE END

Two Childhood Obesity Prevention Programs That Have Actually Been Proven to Work

In the wake of the September 19[th,] 2006 Institute of Medicine report (http://www.iom.edu/Object.File/Master/36/984/11722_reportbrief.pdf) that collectively documents our nation's failure to address the childhood obesity crisis, I'd like to talk about two programs that *have actually been proven to work under real life conditions.*

PE4Life in Naperville, IL

The first, PE4Life, is a well organized, well funded, and scientifically documented project whose model program flourishes at Madison Junior High, School District # 203 in Naperville, IL. PE4Life in Naperville is headed up by Phil Lawler, former physical educator and coach who now serves as the Director of the PE4Life Academy, an affiliated project that's designed to show interested physical educators and educational administrators from around the nation how Madison Junior High's PE4Life program works.

Only Three Percent of Our Kids are Obese...

In School District # 203 only 3% of their students are obese. Compare that to over 15% nationally, and you'll see why decision makers from around the nation are flocking to Lawler's PE4Life Academy to find out what he knows that the rest don't know. "We've trained people from forty different states and five foreign countries," observed Lawler. "I'd say that's a pretty good indicator of the interest levels in this program, wouldn't you agree?"

Corporate Sponsors

PE4Life can boast of corporate sponsors including companies like Reebok, Asics, Gatorade, Quaker Oats, Life Fitness, and Dick's Sporting Goods just to name a few (http://www.pe4life.org/sponsors.php). And anyone visiting Madison Junior High will be blown away by the cutting edge training equipment that Lawler has attracted to this program. "In all honesty, there are NFL, NBA, and MLB trainers who would be green with envy if they saw the equipment that we have," Lawler said. "In a very real sense Madison Junior High is the Mecca for kid's fitness in America today."

For Example...

For example, when MJH students hustle in at the end of gym class, it's common to see every student in class placing his or her Polaris heart rate monitor back in its appropriate location before heading off to the showers. "Polaris has graciously provided us with enough heart rate monitors to cover every student in class. And with the help of these devices, our kids learn all about their own cardiovascular system, and how exercise affects it," Lawler said.

Each student works with this kind of equipment several times a week and they learn about fitness in a very hands-on way. "When they graduate from high school they'll have all the info necessary to keep themselves fit for the rest of their life," said Lawler.

The PE4Life curriculum takes its students beyond cardio fitness, venturing into strength development, agility, quickness, and flexibility. So it's not only the high tech, 21st century characteristics that distinguish this unique program apart from almost everything else in the nation. It's *the cutting edge comprehensiveness* that makes it stand out.

The PE4Life Academy

There are good reasons why physical educators and educational administrators travel great distances to see, hear, taste, smell, and touch what Lawler's students are doing. And that hands-on informational experience is called the PE4Life Academy.

"I get calls from some of the top professors in some of America's top colleges and universities who come from various parts of the nation in order to see what our kids are doing differently here in District #203. We've worked hard for over a decade to bring this program to life, and I think it's safe to say that our entire community takes pride in what our kids have accomplished. It's one of those things that distinguishes Naperville and makes it such a great place to live."

More Than a Childhood Obesity Prevention Strategy

I reality PE4Life is much more than just a childhood obesity prevention strategy. It's a fully equipped, fully funded, comprehensive kid's fitness project whose most eloquent claim to fame is that it's been tested under real world circumstances, and it has proven to be effective. And in a world full of hand wringing and theoretical talk, projects that actually work tend to stand out. For a full explanation check out the PE4Life web site at www.PE4Life.com.

Operation Pull Your Own Weight

On the other side of the tracks (literally on the other side of the Mississippi River) sits another childhood obesity prevention program that's also been proven to work. It's called *Operation Pull Your Own Weight (OPYOW)*, and in almost every conceivable way OPYOW is the polar opposite of Naperville's PE4Life.

One Part of an At Risk Grant

OPYOW was developed at Jefferson Elementary School from 1990-1994*, and was originally underwritten by a state of *Iowa At-Risk Grant* that aimed to improve the self esteem and related performances of the kids who attended Jefferson School.

"OPYOW was the physical component of the self esteem recipe that we were asked to develop," said former Jefferson School Principal Henry Reams. "It was based on the old gym teacher's observation that *kids who can do pull ups, can't be obese*. So the more Jefferson students who learned to pull their own weight, the fewer we'd have doing battle with obesity and related issues. And as we all know, obesity drags a kids self esteem down faster than anything you can think of," said Reams.

Financing OPYOW With Spare Change

Although the grant covered the salaries and related expenses for four teachers, there was *almost no budget for fitness equipment*, and certainly no corporate sponsors. So Reams and company drove to the local Farm and Fleet, where with pennies from the spare change drawer they financed all the materials required to build *sixteen height adjustable pull up bars* (one for every K-2 classroom in school), the only equipment necessary to implement the program.

They asked an Industrial Arts class at Davenport Central High to cut the pipe and chains to the right length, and the district's maintenance department to install one height adjustable pull up bar in every (sixteen) K-2 classroom in school. "*I know we spent less than $200 dollars* to outfit this entire aspect of the grant. You might say we funded OPYOW on a shoestring, begging, borrowing, and stealing everything we needed to get started. But if you check the results, it's hard to be unimpressed with what our students accomplished," said Reams.

What Were the Results?

So what exactly were the results of OPYOW? Over a four year period, from the fall of 1990 through the spring of

1994 hundreds of Jefferson School students not only developed the ability to do pull ups, but they also *learned to look forward to their opportunity to get on the pull up bar and get stronger day after day*, week after week, and month after month. "I've known lots of kids who want to be bad, but I've never met one that wants to be weak, in any way. And with OPYOW we taught students how to get strong in all kinds of ways," Reams said.

What Else Did They Learn?

What else did Jefferson kids learn in OPYOW you ask? "Our kids learned that given the opportunity, they could tackle a difficult task by working at it regularly, making thin slices of progress over a period of time, and in the end they learned to expect success," Reams said.

Jefferson's students also learned that there are six things that increase your strength on the pull up bar, including…

- regular work
- eating right
- getting enough rest
- avoiding tobacco
- avoiding alcohol
- avoiding drugs

"Interestingly enough, when these same six strength building principles are applied to academics they make kids stronger in reading, writing, and arithmetic too," Reams added.

Nobody Else Can Do It For You

One other thing Jefferson students learned from working on a pull up bar was that nobody else can do the work for you. "On the pull up bar our students learned that *they had to take responsibility for getting their own work done, eating right, getting their rest, and avoiding tobacco, alcohol, and drugs.* If they failed to do these things, the pull up bar knew immediately and denied the public success that all kids crave. It was a real eye opener," Reams said, "and that may be the single most important thing our kids learned from OPYOW."

OPYOW Shortcomings

What are the shortcomings of OPYOW? "The biggest void in the program was that it was built on the anecdotal observation that kids who can do pull ups can't be obese," said Reams. "In other words, to my knowledge nobody has ever compared the BMI's of kids who can do pull ups against kids who can't do pull ups in order to scientifically prove that they're a legitimate antidote to obesity. By the same token nobody has ever tried to prove that your nose is located on your face either. Maybe both are too intuitively obvious to attract academia," he added.

A second criticism of OPYOW claimed that, by virtue of focusing on one exercise alone, *it lacked the comprehensiveness that characterizes all well conceived programs*. "But the people who made those claims failed to see that this program never claimed to be comprehensive. Its only claim was that *it's a functional antidote to obesity*...nothing more, nothing less. If you can do pull ups, you can't be obese. By the same token, to the degree that it successfully discourages obesity, it also reduces the workload on the participant's heart 24/7," Reams said.

What Jefferson School students did prove beyond a shadow of a doubt was that, given the right opportunity, *almost all kids can learn to perform pull ups*. "And to the degree that the old coach's intuition is true, Operation Pull Your Own Weight is the simplest and most efficient childhood obesity prevention strategy anyone ever devised," Reams added with a smile.

PE4Life Shortcomings?

How about shortcomings in PE4Life? This program has all the scientific documentation that anyone could ever want. They have money. They have equipment. They have nice neighborhoods and well funded schools. They have a comprehensive 21st century fitness strategy that successfully combats obesity. And school districts that have plenty of money should definitely check it out and see if PE4Life is the answer to their problems.

Lawler suggests that the stakes are now so high that we can no longer afford to use the excuse that school districts can't afford a viable obesity prevention program. By the same token there are 45,000,000 people in America today who are unable to afford health insurance, and it does little good to tell them that their lack of money is no excuse. They're still unable to afford health insurance no matter how you spin it. Are school districts any different?

Equipment Dependency VS Free Agency

On the other hand, even if your school district is overflowing with funds, the PE4Life orientation tends to produce students who are dependent on the high tech equipment that the program is built around. In other words, without access to expensive, high tech, 21st century fitness equipment, PE4Life has little to offer.

In contrast OPYOW creates students who are dependent on a ten dollar, doorway pull up bar, or the closest tree limb. You could call it Tom and Huck fitness. Their expressed goal is what they call *Free Agency (no dependency),* and they claim that it's Mother Nature's antidote to childhood obesity. Now is anyone suddenly feeling a strong desire for a banana?

Similarities between PE4Life and OPYOW include…

- Both have succeeded under real life (as opposed to theoretical) conditions
- Both put the responsibility for success in the hands of the student
- Both were developed by guys from Iowa
- Both feature life long lessons that are tucked in between the lines

Differences between PE4Life and OPYOW

- PE4Life was built on empirical data, OPYOW was built on common sense
- PE4Life requires plenty of money, OPYOW can be implemented on a shoestring
- PE4Life requires lots of equipment, OPYOW requires a height adjustable pull up bar
- PE4Life requires extensive training, OPYOW can be taught by any parent volunteer

- PE4Life requires lots of space for equipment, OPYOW requires no extra space
- PE4Life requires several hours per week, OPYOW requires five minutes per week
- PE4Life encourages equipment dependency, OPYOW encourages free agency
- PE4Life requires a "professional setting," OPYOW can easily be taught at home
- PE4Life's strength is its comprehensiveness, OPYOW's strength is its simplicity
- PE4Life is more than obesity prevention, but for OPYOW that's the whole enchilada
- PE4Life is alive and kicking, OPYOW ran out of funding over a decade ago

The Choice is Yours

So if you have plenty of money, space, equipment, and time to train your trainers, then PE4Life may be a viable option. On the other hand if your school is short on funds, your teachers are already overloaded to the gills, and you have almost no extra time in your curriculum, then the simplicity of Operation Pull Your Own Weight may be more your cup of tea.

*Despite four years of well documented success, OPYOW has been inactive since the grant ran out in the spring of 1994. But with childhood obesity running rampant, there's a movement afoot to breathe life back into this simple, cost effective, tried childhood obesity prevention strategy that's been proven to work. Check out www.childhood-obesity-prevention.com, and www.pullyourownweight.net. They're in the market for corporate sponsors.

A Letter To The Editor...

Elizabeth Taylor, Editor
Chicago Tribune Magazine

The Secret Solution To Childhood Obesity That All Gym Teachers Already Know About ...

Dear Ms. Taylor:

The continuous hand wringing in the media over what is now being called the epidemic in childhood obesity seems to be reaching fever pitch, with the latest treatment in the April 25th edition of *The Chicago Tribune Magazine* entitled "Child Obesity: What Can We Do?"

I know that multi millions of dollars are being spent to resolve this multi billion dollar problem, and the experts and researchers around the country have offered lots of advice that seems to be making almost no headway at all. In fact the problem just seems to be getting bigger by the week. So in the wake of all this, I thought that a real simple observation from a former gym teacher and coach might be of interest to your readers who want their kids to avoid all the problems associated with childhood obesity.

So here's my *observation number one*. In seventeen years of teaching and coaching at various levels, I noticed that students who could perform pull ups were NEVER OBESE. On the other hand those students who were obese COULD NEVER DO PULL UPS. In other words, obesity and the ability to perform pull ups are mutually exclusive, and are NEVER FOUND IN THE SAME PERSON.

Observation number two is, I also noticed that if you start them young (kindergarten, 1st, 2nd grade), before they've had a chance to pick up much extra weight, THERE ARE VERY FEW KIDS WHO ARE UNABLE TO LEARN TO PERFORM PULL UPS. In fact I have personally taught many hundreds of kids that ability, with very few failures I might add.

Observation number three is that as long as that student maintains the ability to perform pull ups, they will never ever carry much excess body weight, let alone be obese. That means that once a child has been taught to perform pull ups, he or she is ARMED WITH A NATURAL, FUNCTIONAL ANTIDOTE TO OBESITY FOR THE REST OF THEIR LIVES, if they choose to maintain that ability. That is to say they are effectively *immunized and vaccinated against obesity forever,* by maintaining the simple and natural ability to do pull ups.

Now if you're tired of waiting for the experts to come up with the magic pill that some pharmaceutical company can manufacture and sell for big bucks, maybe you'd be interested in the advice of a former gym teacher who says that no matter how old you are, if you learn to perform pull ups, you have to be pretty lean. Furthermore, the more pull ups you can do, the leaner you have to be...naturally.

So, if you've seen what I, and *every other gym teacher in the nation* has seen, the solution to childhood obesity is just not all that difficult. Let's teach kids, starting at a very young age, to perform pull ups, and before you know it, childhood obesity will be in the rear view mirror instead of in the headlines of the Tribune. And if your readers have comments or questions I'd love to hear them and answer them.

Sincerely,

Rick Osbourne
Former Physical Educator
Osbourne@chilitech.com
Lombard, IL 60148

Disclaimer OPYOW

We fully recognize that <u>all exercises in which the participant's own body weight is the primary resistance factor</u> (functional work) benefit from fat loss (an excess workload reduction). That is to say, exercise activities such as push ups, sit ups, squats, dips, pull ups, hand stand push ups jumping jacks, squat thrusts, walking, running, dancing, stair climbing will all improve with fat loss.

Not All Body Weight Exercises Qualify

However not all body weight exercises can predictably distinguish people who are obese apart from people who are not obese. In order to do that the body weight exercise must be sufficiently challenging.

So for example jumping jacks don't qualify as predictors of obesity because some or many obese people can do jumping jacks. Dips on the other hand do qualify because those who can do them, can't be obese. Sit ups don't qualify, but hand stand push ups do. Stair climbing doesn't qualify, but pull ups do. In general, the more challenging the exercise, the more qualified and valuable it becomes as a predictor of obesity.

Another Variable

On the other hand, just because a participant is unable to perform pull ups, dips, or hand stand push ups doesn't mean they're obese. It's entirely possible for a person to be skinny, weak, and lack the strength to do these kinds of challenging exercises. But people who are able to perform them are relatively lean and strong.

Here's Why We Chose Pull Ups

The main point here is, *we're not claiming that pull ups have any corner on this functional acid test (FAT) orientation to obesity prevention*. But they're certainly one good example of it. The reason we chose pull ups over all the others are threefold. First, most people know what pull ups are. Second, pull ups are inevitably associated with strength. And third, they line up so perfectly with the phrase Pull Your Own Weight.

Other Virtues

Other distinct virtues of pull ups include the fact that they're extremely affordable, they require very little space to perform, and done right they're infinitely measurable. But if someone wanted to substitute dips, hand stand push ups, or a seven minute mile in place of pull ups, you'd get no argument out of us at all.

A Guarantee...
To Kids Around The World

If you do what I suggest, you'll earn your way onto wall A, a place where all members are lean and strong. Once you get there however, it's up to you to stay there. In other words once you've developed the ability, it's up to you to continue Pulling Your Own Weight.

How To Win Their Hearts...

"Do you know how to win a five year old boy's heart? Well, you drop down to one knee, look him right in the eye, and listen as if what he's telling you is really important...cause it is. And if you happen to speak at all, whatever you say from that position will be infinitely better than anything you can possibly say from on high. Oh, and by the way, five year old girls? They're just the same."
...A wise old coach somewhere, sometime, someplace

www.ingramcontent.com/pod-product-compliance
Lightning Source LLC
Chambersburg PA
CBHW051231050326
40689CB00007B/875